SKIN FITNESS

WITHDRAWN

SKIN FITNESS

Safe and healthy skin care

HUGH MOLLOY & GARRY EGGER

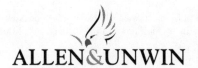

ALLEN&UNWIN

First published in 2008

Allen & Unwin
83 Alexander Street
Crows Nest NSW 2065
Australia
Phone: (61 2) 8425 0100
Fax: (61 2) 9906 2218
Email: info@allenandunwin.com
Web: www.allenandunwin.com

National Library of Australia
Cataloguing-in-Publication entry:

Molloy, Hugh, 1930– .
    Skin fitness : safe and healthy skin care.

    Includes index.
    ISBN 978 1 74175 373 8 (pbk.).

    1. Skin - Care and hygiene. 2. Lifestyles - Health aspects.
    3. Environmental health. 4. Skin - Diseases. 5.
    Dermatopharmacology. I. Egger, Garry. II. Title.

    646.726

Typeset in 10/14 pt Minion by Midland Typesetters, Australia
Printed in Australia by McPherson's Printing Group, Maryborough

10 9 8 7 6 5 4 3 2 1

CONTENTS

FOREWORD TO FIRST EDITION

Much of the impulse for this book came from a single appearance Hugh Molloy made on ABC Radio National's *Health Report*. After he put forward his ideas and findings, the phone, as they say, melted. We had more requests for tapes and transcripts than we had ever had and it was clear that these concepts about skin care had induced a mass 'Aha!' reaction.

When the word 'lifestyle' is used, most of us don't think about our skin. Nor do we usually consider our largest organ when the environment is mentioned.

This is an eco-skin book but it's not about the loss of forests or the large scale environment. Hugh Molloy's theories, supported by his and others' research, are that our micro-environment, the hotel room we find ourselves in, the clothes we wear and exercise in, the bedding we use and poke out of, sweating and itching, how we wash—these factors affect the condition of our skin.

If we already have a propensity for certain skin diseases, an adverse micro-environment can make them worse or harder to treat.

Hugh is very careful to say that he doesn't cure anything. This book isn't a quick fix but it does offer ways of minimising your problems and perhaps at times reducing the need for medication.

And I can tell you that Hugh practises what he preaches. You're hard put to find soap at his place and there's not a doona in sight.

See what you think.

Dr Norman Swan,
Presenter of ABC Radio's *Health Report* and
Walkley Award-winning journalist

ABOUT THE AUTHORS

DR HUGH MOLLOY MRCS (Eng), LRCP (Lond), DObst RCOG (Eng), DDM (Syd), FACD

Hugh Molloy completed his basic medical education at the University of Sheffield in England. Following some years of hospital work he was a ship's surgeon for three and a half years before practising as a GP in Queensland for ten years, an environment which led him to specialist training in Dermatology. Dr Molloy has been a visiting specialist and consultant at a number of adult's and children's teaching hospitals in Sydney and has carried out research in heat studies at Oxford University, where he became an Honorary Consultant to the Department of Dermatology. He is currently retired from practice, living in Sydney.

DR GARRY EGGER MPH PhD MAPS

Garry Egger has qualifications in behavioural biology and public health. He has spent almost four decades in health promotion in government, industry and as a consultant for the World Health Organization (WHO) throughout Australia, Asia and the Pacific. He is the author of over 100 scientific articles and 26 books, including five texts. More recently, Dr Egger was the Developer and Scientific Director of the GutBusters men's 'waist loss' program (more recently 'Professor Trim's Weight Loss Program for Men') and teaches 'Lifestyle Medicine' to doctors throughout Australia. He is Director of the Centre for Health Promotion and Research in Sydney and an Adjunct Professor of Health Sciences at Deakin, Southern Cross and Newcastle Universities.

• • •

SUE PLATER

Sue Plater has been a regular cartoonist for several health publications over the past fifteen years. She has a Graduate Certificate in Health Promotion and works in Aboriginal health for the Queensland Department of Health.

INTRODUCTION

This is a book about skin; more specifically, it's about common skin problems of our time and their possible causes and management. It was never meant to solve, or even discuss, *all* the different types of disorders related to the skin. We haven't pretended to look at infectious skin diseases, or even those with internal origins. Instead, we've tried to encourage a new way of thinking about the causes of many common skin problems related to lifestyle and the modern environment, and to highlight what can be done, by you, to redress them. In particular, we have identified and offered solutions to three of the most common, and yet generally unrecognised, causes of a wide range of skin problems seen in practice today. These are simply:

- overheating
- excessive dryness (xerosis) and
- our modern obsession with cleanliness and technology.

It is our contention that these three factors, alone and/or in combination, are responsible for a large proportion of modern skin problems ranging from certain forms of eczema and psoriasis, to persistent forms of acne. Yet, they have all but been ignored in skin care education in favour of commercial advertising that promotes

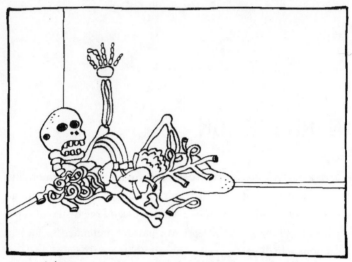

WHAT WE WOULD LOOK LIKE WITHOUT OUR SKIN.

skin products which, in many cases, have the potential to worsen the conditions they claim to 'cure'.

Our thesis is that with skin problems much of what happens, as in many other areas of health in modern society (heart disease, obesity, cancers and injury), results from our way of life rather than any mysterious or unknown microbes of the 21st century. And while this is not meant to deny the huge advances in our modern standards of living, it is meant to sound a warning: that we must not ignore the downside of economic and technological progress when discussing human health.

If you think this sounds a bit radical and not applicable to you, check the list of potential problems related to these three factors in the 'skindex' below:

A 'skindex' of skin and associated problems

A list of modern skin problems with a possible lifestyle cause:

1. Dry, rough or scaly skin which may or may not be itchy.
2. Redness, greasiness, rashes, persistent acne with no obvious cause.
3. Limp, lifeless, stringy or greasy hair.
4. Dark, baggy rings around the eyes ('doona eyes').
5. Comedones ('whiteheads/blackheads') on the forehead, cheeks and chin.
6. Redness and itchiness between the breasts.
7. Recurrent tinea pedis.
8. Unexplained morning sneezing, blocked/dry nose, dry throat.
9. Disturbed sleep.
10. Feeling tired/washed out on waking.

If you suffer any of these at any time, check the behaviour list below to see if any of the following could be a potential cause:

Skin behaviour checklist

Do you:

- try to stay as warm as possible at all times?
- work in an airconditioned office?
- drive an airconditioned car?
- sleep with a doona and/or electric blanket, heated waterbed/tracksuit at night?
- shampoo your hair daily or every two days?
- frequently use soap, deodorant, astringents, exfoliant, aftershave, tonics or toners?

- regularly stay in hotels/motels without external ventilation?
- travel regularly in aeroplanes?
- work, play or lie in the sun?

Most of the problems listed in the 'skindex', as well as a range of related skin problems, are more likely to have a lifestyle basis than any exotic explanation, despite the fact that you've probably never been told so. The purpose of this book is to explain how and why.

1 Why a book on skin and the environment?

Search through the Internet on 'skin', and you'll find hundreds of thousands, possibly millions, of entries. Open these and you'll invariably find an ad for a skin care product. If you just want information about the skin, you're bound to be directed to one or other of these products. It's difficult to find any impartial source of information on how to look after or manage your skin which doesn't involve you buying something (probably very expensive) or undergoing some equally expensive treatment guaranteed to 'promote rejuvenation'.

The skin care market is big business. It's estimated at well over $1 billion per year in Australia (excluding cosmetics) and is the most rapidly growing division of the pharmaceutical industry worldwide. At least 25 per cent of all medical consultations involve the skin, and of these an estimated 75 per cent are due to personal mismanagement of the skin to some degree. Many problems come from the treatments initially aimed at making the problem better. They are 'iatrogenic', which means literally 'caused by the treatment'. But a lot of skin problems also come from what we consider to be a more important but less obvious cause—the modern environment, both personal and communal.

Of course, not all skin problems are entirely environmentally related. So by definition this book is not meant to cover all skin disorders. Certain types of problems need to be looked at by a specialist. But the proposal we'll expound here, and one that's reinforced by a growing number of skin problems in industrialised societies, is that much of the damage done to our skin in modern times results from our environment and our personal behaviour. In our desire for perfection, as encouraged by the social pressures of the time, we tend to *over*-cleanse, *over*heat and *over*-medicate our bodies, and this often is expressed as problems of the skin, which today are more prominent than in previous times. For those with no current skin damage, the information we present here is, at the very least, likely to protect your skin against future damage and make you feel more comfortable. For those with existing problems, it could provide a new approach on the road to recovery.

Skin through the ages

Skin keeps us in. It manufactures vitamins and hormones and it translates the 'inner' messages of the body to the outer world and makes us aware of what is going on around us. It has served the same functions through half a million years of evolution. And although times may have changed, the basic functions of human skin have not. Humans have undoubtedly suffered skin problems, generally referred to throughout this book as 'dermatitis' (see Chapter 4), throughout history. But can you imagine thousands of Dreamtime Aborigines with zits? Or vast hoards of Aztec warriors with acne?

Why is it that we seem to have so many and such diverse skin problems today, in an era when so many 'scientific' or 'clinically proven' skin treatments are available? Why do we worry so much about body odour when there's a pharmacopoeia of deodorants, from animal glands to flower scent, available? Most body odour comes from wearing unwashed clothing for days and days. Many patients, when closely questioned, will admit to changing their

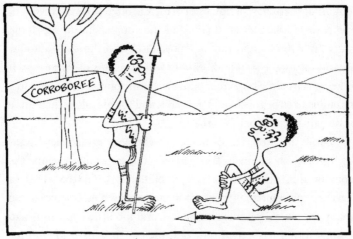

"I CANT GO. I'VE GOT A ZIT."

outer clothing regularly, but making their underwear 'last a little longer'! Why do we feel so dirty, greasy and itchy when every Australian uses, on average, 21 bars of soap a year? (Interestingly, the figures for the United Kingdom are 4–6, and for France 1–2.) A cynic would be forgiven for thinking that if any product was truly successful, skin problems would have disappeared, rather than grown to the multi-billion dollar industry the cosmetics game is today.

Something happened to our skin on the way to the second millennium. It's to do with the environment and our personal behaviour. It's to do with economic growth. It's to do with technology and its effects on the modern environment. There's no doubt technology has been good to us. It has provided us with effort-saving devices such as cars, washing machines, vacuum cleaners and central heating, and entertainment—mainly of a passive type—like TV, videos, remote controls and the Internet.

But all of these have a downside which is often not recognised in the rush for the eternal dollar and the compulsion to be 'doing something more important or enjoyable'. The technology of today is paid for by the skin and other health problems of tomorrow. It takes at least ten days to reorganise a routine physical response to a stimulus or to begin changing a habit, and the old adage that 'there is no gain without pain' is true.

While the problems of modern technology are acknowledged by most health scientists, there's little scope for profit in selling the complications of the technological revolution—the fact that we might have too much airconditioning, too many household chemicals, too many cosmetics, too much rich food, and too little opportunity to exercise is not recognised. The purpose of this book is to examine those aspects of our modern environment that may be causing or contributing to some of the skin problems of today, and which we may be able to change without too much interference with our daily life. We don't intend to suggest a 'quick fix' or a pill to cure your skin problems overnight. *Most skin change is slow.* No one can give you a new skin—even the best laser in town is incapable of doing this. However, we can give you some understanding, in simple terms, of what your skin is, how it works, how it reacts to what you do, and what you can do to get the most out of what you have been given.

Our aim is to show you how to care for your skin using simple, relatively inexpensive aids. As you'll see, this could also result in saving you a small fortune—in money and time. The only expensive item will be in effort and commitment on your part. You will have to do most of the work. In doing this we'll bear in mind the following quotation by Hippocrates: 'First of all, do no harm.'

No advice we give here could possibly be considered dangerous or invasive. Our main objective is to help you avoid cumulative damage to the skin. Where complicated internal medical conditions, genetic disorders, abnormal immunological/biochemical disorders, cancer, or systemic infections are involved, more specific advice and treatment should be sought. Some of these will no doubt have adverse effects upon the skin. There will need to be a trade-off. Even so, the simple guidelines suggested here—and they are very simple—will serve only to enhance the effects of that treatment.

• • •

As already mentioned, the message of this book is that many modern skin problems come directly from the environment and our personal behaviour. Our desire to always stay warm, to be meticulously clean, to have hair like the film stars and to look forever young is leading us to overuse airconditioning, bedding, soaps and shampoos, mindlessly ignorant of any potential consequences. Dermatologists are beginning to recognise this, as demonstrated by the fact that in 1998 a whole issue of the journal *Clinical Dermatology* was devoted to environmental dermatology, looking particularly at man-made environments. As noted in that issue, '. . . a large percentage, if not the majority of modern skin problems (in contrast to skin diseases), come from the environment and our personal behaviour'.

The use of scientific and clinical evidence

One of the key achievements of the modern age has been scientific discovery. If a relationship is mooted between a pathogen and a disease, it can be put to the test. The more times it is tested and proven, the more likely there is to be an association. In science, this is known as Koch's Postulates, after the philosopher and physician Joseph Koch (1846–1910).

Unfortunately, in recent times a tendency has developed to reduce all observations to a series of numbers so that they may be more 'scientifically analysed'—this is known as evidence-based medicine. While this may have advantages, we wonder whether the trend has gone too far, and we have lost the benefits of past wisdom.

Cosmetics manufacturers and skin product marketers use the term 'scientifically proven' with great abandon. And while the true use of proper scientific evidence is to be applauded, there is enough misinterpretation of the facts to make the public sceptical. On the other hand, much evidence comes from clinical practice and physiological understanding. Although some may not consider this to be truly 'scientific', it can give a clue to relationships which may be then tested. In our case, we hope that the combination of our experience in science, clinical practice and epidemiology will help us keep an even balance throughout the book.

Skin 'fitness'

The major issues with which we are concerned here are dry ('non-waterproofed') skin, the effects of sweat entrapment in the outer layer of the skin and the ways in which this is facilitated by the modern environment. This combination can precipitate and perpetuate a great variety of skin reactions. There are six major factors involved:

1. **'Dry' skin.** This is not a very satisfactory term. Instead, we've generally used the terms 'waterproofed' and 'non-waterproofed' skin. Dry skin is difficult to document or to measure accurately and inexpensively. But most people recognise it from a feeling of roughness. Perhaps the majority of people have inherited dry skin and this is a risk factor for further skin damage. There are some genetic markers of dry skin, easily detected in a simple physical examination.

2. **Climate.** Australia is well recognised as having a very dry climate, and this is likely to get drier in many parts with the advent of climate change. Along the southeast coastline, the daily variations in temperature and humidity can be as great as almost anywhere else in the world. Australia also suffers from prolonged droughts, and at times the bushfire ratings remain high for long periods, indicating dry earth, dry vegetation, dry air and dry skin. Although cities such as Sydney are seen as having a humid climate, in comparison with other parts of the world all of Australia is dry.

3. **Airconditioning and certain forms of heating.** Air is dried out by reverse-cycle airconditioners and heaters (gas and slow-combustion heaters, and heaters containing fans). The relative humidity in the average large passenger plane can get down as low as 3 per cent on a long flight. Optimum relative humidity on the other hand, and that with which skin is most comfortable, lies in the mid range, between 40 and 65 per cent. However, as long as the relative humidity is less than 100 per cent, there will be a net outward diffusion of water from the lower layers of the skin which, under certain circumstances, can lead to skin drying. Modern airconditioning in homes, planes, cars and offices is one of the main drying factors in the environment.

4. **The overuse of soaps and shampoos (industrial detergents).** These wash the natural greases (or waterproofing) out of the stratum corneum, or the barrier layer of the skin (see next chapter). In doing so, they dry the skin and expose it to external irritants and

the exigencies of internal factors. The more cleansing and detergent-like the soap or shampoo, the greater its drying and scouring effect, resulting in the very thing these products are meant to protect from: dehydrated and vulnerable skin.

5. **Other environmental factors**. Sun, salt water and chlorinated water all have some beneficial effect on the skin. But they can also dry it out and thus damage the barrier layer of skin, which is the main protective layer between you and the external environment. Frequently used cosmetics, toners, tonics, facial cleansers, astringents, exfoliants or aftershave lotions can add to this damage through the cumulative effects of excessive drying (see Chapter 5). Smooth skin is very attractive, but it can hide dryness.

    'Any surface you admire for its function or its beauty should be polished.' Bacteria find it very difficult to flourish on shiny surfaces. This is why you polish your dining room table. You can then pick up a piece of bread or a biscuit and eat it without first having to wash it or dip it in antiseptic!

6. **Overheating at night or in bed**. When humans are exposed to cold, it takes only minutes for this to be noticed. Warming up the body, on the other hand, is gradual and can occur almost without awareness, particularly during sleep, when it takes two to three hours. For this reason most people overheat in bed— even when sleeping alone! The invention of efficient insulation for buildings, heating for cars and synthetic clothing to keep us warm have also contributed to the

situation of overheating. The reduction in our naturally acquired immunity to a wide variety of infections, both major and minor, probably due in some part to the widespread use of antibiotics, has fostered the idea that we're more likely to 'catch something nasty' if we don't keep warm. This applies particularly to children. While heat and warmth *per se* are not problems for the human body, a lack of experience with variations in temperature and the drying effects of prolonged heating, if not countered in some way by proper skin care, can become a big problem (see Chapter 5).

The 'take-home' messages

Based on the above factors, there are a number of ' take-home' messages from this book which may, at first glance, appear startling. Some of these include the facts that:

- overheating at night through the use of a doona, continental quilt or artificial heating in bed can cause problems with scalp and hair, itchy eyes with pigmentation ('doona eyes'), facial dermatitis and persistent 'acne-like' eruptions;
- far from giving you beautiful shiny hair as in the ads, the overuse of shampoo can actually damage your hair and make it dry and lifeless;
- the detergent effects of shampoo around the feet in the shower might lead to totally unexpected problems such as tinea;
- excessive use of soap and over-showering can aggravate skin problems and increase the perceived need for a deodorant, which in turn may cause a 'dermatitis';

- antiperspirants and deodorants are not necessary for a 'nice' smell and in fact may cause 'dermatitis'/allergic problems;
- toners, tonics, astringents, exfoliants and cleansers can do more harm than good to the skin;
- aftershave and other alcohol-based astringents may smell nice but do little for the skin;
- your office airconditioning could also be damaging your skin.

Amongst other things, we'll be suggesting some ways to help improve your skin such as:

- using blankets instead of a doona, even in the middle of winter—it is difficult to 'peel off' half a doona if one gets too hot;
- avoiding soaps and shampoos to help avoid the need for deodorants;
- using hair conditioner only, instead of shampoo;
- drying long hair with a chamois from the car-parts shop;
- not using baby powder—even on babies!
- losing fat (not necessarily weight);
- 'patting' yourself dry after showering, not 'rubbing';
- using a simple moisturiser *all over* at least once a day (men and women);
- getting used to not always being warm (comfortable is good);
- having tepid (comfortably warm), not very hot, showers;
- punching holes in the insteps of all your leather shoes;
- leaving the bath full of water in your hotel room at night;

- using the windows in your car rather than the airconditioning—and using a fine spray/mist of water through the car regularly on long trips.

At first glance, none of these might seem likely to solve your particular skin problem. But as you will see, treatment (and prevention) depends on cause. Once we begin to understand the causes of many modern skin problems—and see how there is often a common underlying basis—the solution becomes more obvious. Each of the steps outlined above will be considered in detail in the following chapters.

2 Structure of the skin

Before we look at common skin problems, and the best ways to deal with these, it is appropriate to look at just what makes up skin, in simple terms, so we can understand how this may be affected by external factors.

Skin anatomy

Diagram 2.1 shows the basic structure of the skin. There are two main layers: the epidermis on the outside and the dermis underneath. The dermis lies on a bed of subcutaneous fat, backed by a layer of strong fibrous tissue, the deep fascia ('glad wrap'), which encapsulates the whole of the body.

The epidermis arises from a layer of basal cells, which sit on the *basement membrane* that separates the epidermis from the dermis—also known as the *dermo-epidermal junction*. The basal cells grow larger and then divide into two. One half then starts to move in the direction of the surface, becoming known as a *keratinocyte*. The other half stays at the base to complete a number of further cycles. Normal progression of the keratinocyte to the surface takes around 28 days. During this journey it undergoes many complicated physical and chemical changes collectively known as *keratinisation*. Any disorder of this process is referred to as a *dyskeratosis*, most of which are acquired as a result of some form

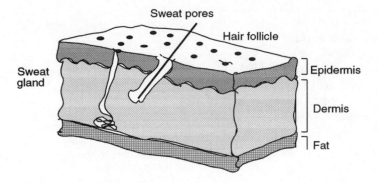

Diagram 2.1 Basic structure of the skin

of external injury or internal disorder, but the more severe forms are due to genetic variations.

Interspersed between the basal cells are *melanocytes*, or pigment-producing cells. These cells produce and package *melanin*, the pigment which is responsible for skin colour. The production of melanin is stimulated by ultraviolet light, hormones, inflammation and injury. The melanin is packaged in *melanosomes* (small 'packages' in the light-skinned races, larger packages in the dark-skinned races) which are passed along very fine tubes (*dendrites*) into the keratinocytes (see diagram 2.2), resulting in variations in skin colour from time to time as a transient tan. It is carried to the surface by the progressing keratinocytes and eventually cast off. Excessive pigment production is followed by some of the pigment 'falling through' the basement membrane to be deposited in the upper dermis, and then being very slowly removed over a number of years by *macrophages*, or scavenger cells.

Also scattered throughout the epidermis are *antigen presenting cells* which function like an early warning system in detecting the presence of noxious substances, bacteria, viruses, parasites

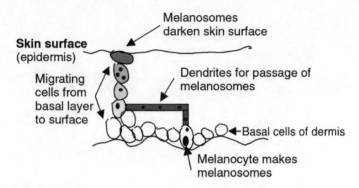

Diagram 2.2 The process of skin darkening by melanin production and distribution

and allergens, alerting the defence (immune) system to initiate a suitable counterattack.

Hair

Specialised down growths of the epidermis into the dermis are directed to the formation of specific skin appendages such as hair follicles, grease glands, sweat glands and nails (see diagram 2.3). Hair serves as a physical protector for the epidermis and as a means of insulating the skin. In areas where there's likely to be a lot of sweating, such as the head, the groin and the armpits, it helps to hold and prevent loss of sweat, allowing it to evaporate and cool the skin locally. Each hair follicle has a tiny muscle (the *arrector pili*) attached to it and this contracts in times of cold, fear or threat, making the hair stand up straight and causing 'goose bumps' at the surface of the skin where the hair follicle opens. This slows down the passage of air over the surface of the skin and helps in the maintenance of warmth. It also exaggerates the aggressive appearance of animals in times of conflict, giving the message to their rivals, 'do not mess with me'.

Hair in humans, and its equivalent of feathers in birds, is also important in the sexual display of both males and females, the peacock's fan being a good example. In humans, this may explain the massive attention given to hair care and presentation by commercial marketers, and the potential side effects of this as we discuss later in Chapter 7.

Why do we have hair?

Sweat is only effective if it can be cooled by the surrounding air. Sweat that drops off the body does not have this effect and is thus wasted in the cooling process. Hence there are several parts of the body where sweat is designed to be held, rather than to drop off the body, until such time as it can be evaporated locally. Increased hair in areas of high sweat production—on the scalp, eyebrows, armpits, lower back, groin and the pubic region—has this effect in preventing run-off of sweat and consequent lack of evaporative cooling.

Sweat

Sweat comes from the *eccrine* sweat glands, as shown in diagram 2.3. These secrete a clear, slightly odorous fluid (sweat), the main function of which is to evaporate on the skin surface to prevent overheating. Another function of sweat, particularly in the palms of the hands and soles of the feet, is to help us to hold on more tightly to objects in our grasp, particularly in situations of fear. Sweat on the body is occurring, to some degree, all the time and hence the eccrine glands are a most important part of body function helping to maintain the constant state of the body's metabolism.

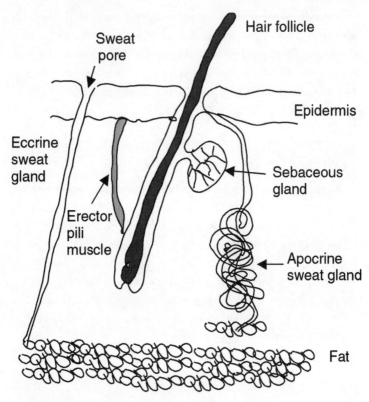

Diagram 2.3 The body's cooling system

Life without sweating is very difficult. At rest, with no visible perspiration, the loss from the eccrine sweat glands is about 300–500ml per day, much of which is from the palms of the hands and the soles of the feet. Under very hot conditions (e.g. during a long run), as much as 2 litres per hour may be lost as sweat. The fact that sweat contains some urea is interpreted by some people as a secondary way of excreting nitrogen from the body, but it's probably

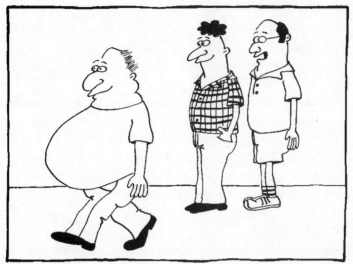

"HE'S CALLED 'SKINNY' BECAUSE HE HAS MORE SKIN THAN MOST."

that the urea is present because it helps in the better hydration of the stratum corneum.

Another type of gland shown in diagram 2.3 is the *apocrine gland* which exists mainly in the armpits, groin and aureole of the nipple. These secrete fluids containing *pheromones*, which are thought to play a part in sexual attraction, and bonding between mother and baby. Recent work has indicated that pheromones may play a part in the regulation of the menstrual cycle and even in ovulation. They have been suggested as a reason for the not infrequent horse-bite injury of the breast sustained by some females during the grooming of their favourite horses. In animals, pheromones cause sexual excitement, provide communication about food and warn other animals in the species about danger. In humans, these functions seem to be less important because we have a sophisticated level of verbal communication. But the extent to which they can still have an influence on our behaviour is not clear.

Sebaceous gland

The *sebaceous gland*, or the third type of gland shown in diagram 2.3, produces a greasy substance from the dead cells within it which grow from the lining of the gland. It helps to keep the skin 'greased', and after puberty acts as a mild antibacterial, antifungal dressing. The sebaceous glands are under partial hormonal control and are the focus of inflammation occurring in acne spots.

Barrier function

Probably the most important part of the epidermis is the stratum corneum—the outermost layers—which form the ultimate barrier between us and our environment. This will be discussed in greater detail later. Suffice to say at this point that the maintenance of adequate hydration (waterproofing) of the stratum corneum can determine the extent of subsequent skin damage.

Dermis

The dermis represents the main structure of the skin. It weighs about one-sixth of the total body weight, and varies in thickness from about 1mm on the face to 4mm on the back. It carries most of the services of the skin. It supplies nutriment to the epidermis and skin appendages, and helps cushion against mechanical injury. The dermis consists of a mixture of substances called *ground substance*, and two specific protein substances, *collagen* and *elastin*, which are manufactured on the spot by cells called *fibroblasts*. These three substances hold an enormous quantity of water in the dermis, giving it a rubbery texture and function.

How does skin 'crack'?

When skin is soft and supple, it bends when pressure is applied, just like a normally ripened tomato. On the other hand, if the skin dries out openings can occur between surface skin cells and these can 'crack' open, like an overripe tomato with force applied to it. This is why big people with dry skin on the heels and feet tend to get 'cracked' skin on the heels when wearing thongs or shoes over which the heel protrudes.

Scattered throughout this watery mixture are other cells such as *mast* (factory) cells, which produce many of the messenger and function chemicals such as *histamine* in response to foreign substances entering the body and causing allergic reactions. In addition we find macrophages (garbage collectors), melanocytes and some white cells (*leucocytes*) which are part of the immune (defence) system. At various levels, usually parallel to the surface, there are networks of blood vessels, lymphatic ducts and nerves with specialised nerve endings, with occasional interconnections between the networks.

Fat

Below the dermis is where we store most of our body fat, which is called *subcutaneous* (below the skin) fat (see diagram 2.1). The thickness and type of fat varies much between the sexes, between families and races and from person to person. It's this which is responsible for soft curvaceous body outlines. It also plays an important part in thermal insulation and protection from blunt external injury.

Deep fascia

The deep fascia is the tissue which holds all the parts of the body together. It forms a capsule around muscles, joints and organs like a type of 'glad wrap' which acts as a protective layer keeping parts of the body in place. The deep fascia is important in the mechanism of pumping the venous blood from the feet up the legs and back to the general circulation. It is also the structure on which the skin facade of the body hangs.

It's amongst this mixture of widely varying tissue that things can go wrong, resulting in problems seen, or felt, in the outer layer of the skin. Knowing how this combination of tissues works when in peak condition or under adverse conditions will help us to understand common skin problems.

3 Function of the skin

The skin is the largest organ of the body (although fat and muscle are now challenging for this title). In the average adult, skin is approximately the size of a 3 x 4 metre carpet. In keeping with its large size is its diversity of function. On a grand scale, it 'keeps us together' and stops us leaking out all over the place. It's also very important in maintaining the internal environment, or *'milieu interior'*. Conversely, it's the first line of defence against the onslaughts of the external environment—wind and rain, variations in temperature and humidity, sunlight and attack from all manner of noxious assailants: physical, chemical, animal, vegetable and organismal (parasitic, fungal, bacterial and viral). In all the above functions, the barrier layer, or layer of the skin which is closest to the outside environment, is the major player.

The skin plays a big part in defining our individuality. It is the major component of our external appearance. It helps us to communicate with the rest of the world at both the conscious and subconscious levels (blushing is just one example of this). It is also capable of acting as a distress flag, giving us a warning that all is not well inside. If there's an internal infection or inflammation, the skin can become hot, red, sore, tender or swollen. If the liver is not functioning properly, or if we are suffering from certain types of anaemia, it may become yellow. It will get itchy in the presence

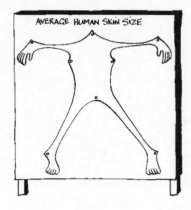
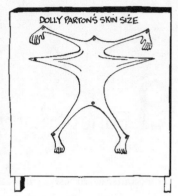

of chemicals to which we've become allergic or if we've been bitten by some marauding insect. A chronic itch in older people can also be an early sign of an internal malignancy not yet evident. 'Winter itch' is a relatively common phenomenon resulting from dry winter air made even drier by internal heating. This can occur at any time of the year in artificial environments.

Less obvious roles of the skin include the production of vitamins, such as vitamin D, which is produced by the effects of sunlight on its precursor in the epidermis. *Pheromones*, secreted by the apocrine glands, are derived from the epidermis. Another type of hormone called a *chalone* is also produced in the skin. It is thought to be important in switching on and off the repair mechanisms in the epidermis.

The stratum corneum

The stratum corneum (SC), or outer layer, is generally regarded as the skin's main physical and chemical barrier. The SC is composed of 'dead cells' which, having started from the basal layer and progressed towards the surface, have slowly lost their active nuclei

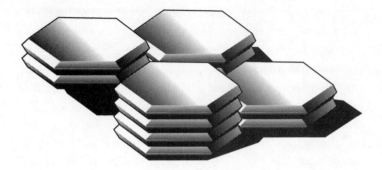

Diagram 3.1 Structure of the skin

and *organelles* (active intracellular factories) and have been filled with resilient protein fibres called *keratin*, laid down in adherent layers, along with some lipid (fatty) substances. They're stacked in columns, interleafing, and attached to each other like bricks in a wall, as shown in diagram 3.1

The spaces between the cells are filled with leaflets of fatty material (lipid and water) known as *inter-cellular cement*. This intimate mixture of grease and water is exceedingly important. Water holds grease and grease holds water. If the delicate balance is upset it leads to problems. As the keratinocytes progress towards the surface, they gradually lose their attachments to each other, eventually being discarded at the surface (*exfoliation*).

The transit of materials—molecules and fluids—both into and out of the body via the skin is not well understood. Three possible routes could be involved: through the cells, between the cells, or via the appendages and glands. It's likely that all three routes are involved, but not equally. It is known, for example, that steroids seem to transit the barrier predominantly through the sebaceous glands, due to their high fat solubility.

Because the dermis can carry up to 25 per cent of the body's blood supply in tiny blood vessels, this offers an effective route for the delivery of drugs through skin 'patches' or subcutaneous injections. The delivery of a few drugs, such as nicotine or hormones from skin patches, is effected by the addition of special transport vehicles enabling the drug to pierce the surface layer of skin. The ability to deliver many drugs in this way is very limited. Despite the claims of many cosmetic manufacturers that creams and lotions containing collagen or elastin—substances which are supposed to break down 'cellulite' (if it truly exists)—can penetrate the skin by simply being rubbed on the outer surface, proof of this is lacking. Most of these substances are not absorbed and have little or no value as an ingredient in a cream. Collagen and elastin can only be effective if produced in the skin by fibroblasts. The apparent random pattern of the networks of such fibres seems to be dependent on the local stresses and strains between the skin and its underlying muscles at a particular site.

Measurement of the traffic into and out of the skin is complicated and not very accurate. Trans-epidermal water and heat loss gives us some idea of the integrity of the barrier, as does the electrical resistance or impedance across it. Radioactive tagging of chemicals placed on or below the skin surface enable us to follow their progress photographically through the barrier, but all of these techniques remain experimental, time consuming and expensive.

The thickness of the stratum corneum varies over the body. There are between ten and twenty layers of cells on average, more in some areas (such as the backs of hands) and less in others (the scrotum and eyelids). In the areas of greatest wear and tear such as the palms of the hands and the soles of the feet, the SC is up to 40 times thicker.

It is generally accepted that the presence of a thin film of grease/oil and water reduces trans-epidermal heat and water loss, and so presumably improves the barrier integrity of the SC in both directions. The guards at Buckingham Palace have known for a long time that the best way to keep their boots in good order is with 'spit and polish'. Well polished or waterproofed skin presents a good barrier to the outside world and influences impinging on it are less able to penetrate the barrier. Un-waterproofed or dry skin, on the other hand, is unable to do this.

Physical, chemical, climatic and allergic influences penetrating the stratum corneum cause non-waterproofed skin to become 'irritable' and more easily insulted. Not only can things penetrate the barrier from the outside, but heat and water vapour are lost more easily from the inside through the surface layer of skin. This is shown graphically in diagram 3.2.

The top-left illustration in diagram 3.2 shows a 'healthy' well hydrated stratum corneum. The surface cells are full of moisture and, as moisture holds grease and grease holds moisture in the cells and between them, they present a solid barrier to the outside world. In the middle illustration, the skin has been dried out and outside influences are able to penetrate either through or between cells. Here, the barrier is compromised, is more easily insulted and can become 'irritable'. The skin reacts to this situation by producing a 'dermatitis', a generic term for any type of inflammatory reaction by the skin to insult (see the next chapter). Long-term insult damages the skin in many ways and makes it a suitable medium for the growth of skin cancer. Short-term insult may just result in itchiness, irritability or redness of the skin which makes life temporarily uncomfortable. Dermatitis of certain types may also become secondarily infected, giving rise to other kinds of skin disorder.

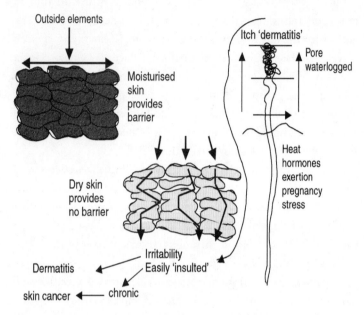

Diagram 3.2 Effects of skin overheating and drying

The right illustration of diagram 3.2 shows sweat ducts which take a spiral course through the epidermis and then proceed downwards as straight ducts to reach the gland in the lower dermis and subcutaneous fat. If the waterproofing has been washed out of the surface layer of skin by the overuse of cleansing products, and increased sweating occurs, the keratin forming the external part of the duct becomes waterlogged and the duct collapses, blocking the flow of sweat to the surface. If sweating continues, the pressure inside the lower part of the duct in the epidermis increases and the sweat may rupture out into the epidermis, where it is recognised as a foreign material and causes an inflammatory reaction. This reaction proceeds to the surface and presents as an 'itch' or 'prickle' or a heat rash, any of which can become a source of further insult to the skin and again cause a 'dermatitis' in the short term, or a more serious problem in the long term.

'Dermatitis' usually results from a multiplicity of factors coming together, rather like the many factors in a road accident. In addition to the six factors mentioned in Chapter 1, there may be other more specific factors, such as irritants or allergens, which can be discovered by examining the lifestyle of the patient prior to the appearance of the rash. Internal factors such as systemic illnesses, drugs and stress and other medical factors also have to be considered. But one of the major neglected precipitants in modern skin disorders is sweat entrapment.

Heat and the skin

The normal functioning of the body is dependent on an underlying metabolism. Metabolism consists of millions of different chemical reactions spread throughout every organ, fuelled by the food we eat and drink and the air we breathe. This immense chemical activity produces energy, any excess of which, in the acute stage, is converted to heat, which slowly seeps out to the surface and thence to the outside world. It does this so the internal environment of the body, the milieu interior, is kept stable within a very small range, around 37 degrees Celsius. Heat is lost from the body, mainly via the skin, from the evaporation of sweat, through convection and radiation. It is also lost to a lesser extent in the air we exhale, and in our urine and faeces. The metabolic rate, and therefore heat production, is controlled by a variety of factors including hormones, the central nervous system, physical activity, emotional states, drugs and even posture.

Sweating

Sweat is secreted by the eccrine sweat glands situated in the lower dermis and subcutaneous fat. It is delivered to the skin surface via sweat ducts (described in Chapter 2) to lie on the surface of the skin until it evaporates into the air, taking up a quantity of heat known as the *latent heat of vaporisation*. When sweat evaporates off the skin (and not until it does so), the body is cooled. Sweat glands are distributed all over the skin, but are found in greater numbers in the *heat-sink* area of the upper torso (from the nipple line to the top of the head), the armpits, the lower back, around the anus and in the groin. Some of these areas are preferentially stimulated by heat, some by stress and some by both of these factors. Sweating can be induced by a range of other factors such as exertion, hormones and pregnancy. Most important, and perhaps most under-rated in terms of its effects on the skin in the modern environment, is sweat created from heat (clothing, artificial heating and exertion).

Radiation and convection

Radiation and convection, the other processes by which heat is lost from the body, can occur from anywhere on the skin surface. Most takes place from the extremities, the hands, feet and head in particular, especially when the rest of the body is clothed. Control of heat loss is mainly associated with the *acral regions*, situated in the fingers, toes, ear lobes and nose. These areas contain specialised neuro-vascular complexes which have the ability to shunt warm arterial blood either to the surface of the skin in order to lose heat, or to the deep tissues of the body in order to conserve heat. If the body is conserving heat, the hands, feet, ear lobes and nose should feel colder than the forehead. This means that the body's thermo-regulatory mechanism is working well, but it takes five minutes at least to stabilise, depending on how well you have trained it. Midriffs do not possess such neuro-vascular complexes, and so do not react to cold so well.

Another means of reducing heat loss when the body is trying to stay warm is the development of goose bumps, caused by the contraction of the erector pili muscles attached to the hair follicles (see diagram 2.3). This causes the hairs to stand up at right angles to the surface, reducing the flow of air across the skin and hence maintaining warmth at the skin surface. It was shown in the 1960s that the detection of cold occurs in the extremities, while overheating is detected centrally in the hypothalamus (lower brain). This may help explain why, particularly during sleep, excess cold is felt within a few minutes, whereas overheating may not be felt for 2 to 3 hours. It's during this lagtime, as we shall see, that damage can be done to the skin.

What are wrinkles and how do they develop?

Wrinkling involves changes in both the epidermis and the dermis, in that both layers become thinner with age, even without exposure to sunlight. This results in the skin becoming thin, fragile, lax and wrinkled, with a tendency to easy bruising. It is exaggerated in the areas of high sunlight exposure. The elasticity of the skin depends on the integrity of the many elastin networks in the dermis. Furrows, which include frown lines, crows feet etc., are due to reshaping of the sheath of elastin which uniquely moulds the facial skin in response to the action of the facial muscles and external forces such as repeated rubbing. In the early stages repair can be induced to some extent by lifestyle changes, but the longer it persists the more permanent it becomes.

Overheating

Overheating results from the weather, artificial heat, too much clothing, or if the cooling mechanisms of the body are paralysed by disease or drugs. In an industrialised society, it is relatively easy to keep warm and warmth can be addictive. Walk into any major store and someone will attempt to sell you something to 'keep you warm'. And yet we live in the subtropics! This is not to deny that it can be cold at night in winter, particularly inland, and in the mountains and the deserts. Yet the Australian climate is overall very mild, even though during the day the temperature and humidity can vary markedly. As a result of this, Australians frequently over-dress in the morning in anticipation of the cold, and by around midday find themselves overheated and unable to divest themselves of some of their numerous layers of clothing. Staying warm has become an expected outcome of our technological society. A degree of warmth gives us solace and comfort. Coming home at the end of a torrid day in the office, feeling that 'nobody loves you', having a drink which gives a warm feeling inside, followed by a warm shower, warm clothing and snuggling up under a warm blanket, with or without a companion, would make anyone feel better. Warmth can be addictive like tobacco, alcohol, heroin and other recreational drugs.

Thermo-regulation and lifestyle

The body's response to the cold (the heat conservation mechanisms referred to above) is usually quick and automatic. If this is inadequate we have to rely on artificial insulation or heating. In response to overheating, there are also control mechanisms which cut in spontaneously. However, in modern society our addiction to warmth can often over-ride these mechanisms. This means that overheating and overdrying of the skin can occur and lead to subsequent skin problems, virtually without our knowing it.

The basic conflict starts with confusion between facts and subjective assessments. We tend to believe that if we feel cold, or if the weather outside looks wintery, the temperature must be low, so we put on extra clothing. We also tend to believe that the insulation capacity of clothing and bed-clothing can be accurately assessed by weight, thickness, feel, fashion and appearance. All these assumptions are incorrect. Whether we feel cold or not depends to a large extent on how well our thermo-regulatory mechanisms have been trained to allow us to adapt to the extremes of hot and cold.

The concept of adaptation is an important one in physiology. It can perhaps best be illustrated in relation to physical fitness. Through regular physical activity, a level of cardiovascular fitness develops in an individual which enables that person to more comfortably operate at the extreme levels of activity. This allows a 'reserve' capacity, such that if you have to run for a bus or away from danger it is possible without too much adverse reaction. The main organ involved in fitness is the heart, and regularly testing the limits of this through exercise helps to maintain it at a level which protects it against such 'insults', which may otherwise cause heart attack. The thermo-regulatory mechanism (TRM) regulates our response to heat and cold via the skin, and unless this is regularly tested to its limits it becomes similarly 'unfit', and less capable of protecting us against environmental variations.

For someone who is regularly exposed to wide ranges of heat and cold, extremes over short periods present no problems. Their 'internal thermostat' is set at a point which is easily accommodated. This is why such people don't 'feel' the cold or the heat as much as someone who is always insulated against the extremes. Someone who is constantly exposed to artificially warm conditions, on the other hand, has a maladjusted TRM which allows overexposure to the ravages of heat and drying and makes any minor level of cold feel unbearable. Hence, where we have set our 'personal thermostat' through regular exposure is important. Like other physical regulatory mechanisms, this will only continue to work well between the limits to which it has recently been tested. For this reason it is important to feel cold from time to time! It is also important to become sensitive to the dangers of overheating, particularly where the body's thermo-regulatory mechanisms may have been dulled into a form of benign acceptance. This doesn't mean we have to roll in the snow or languish in a sauna bath like some supposed health 'gurus' have advocated. But it does suggest that we should be aware of the negative effects of abdicating any changes in sensation made possible through the availability of overly comfortable technology. It's our failure to maintain these natural control mechanisms which can cause skin problems.

Retraining the thermo-regulatory system

Regaining the body's ability to thermo-regulate itself to cope with what may otherwise be seen as uncomfortable levels of cold requires retraining of the body. This necessitates a short period of mild discomfort (like trying to break any form of 'addiction'). About ten nights in winter is usually enough. Going 'cold turkey' means sleeping with a single sheet and cotton blanket, and this might mean waking up several times during the night in the first few nights feeling cold. After rolling over and going back to sleep, however, waking periods will start to decrease and should cease by about night six. After about ten nights sleep should be constant, resulting in a much more refreshed feeling in the morning. This may sound masochistic and does not have a strong research base, but from a clinical perspective it appears to be the most effective way to re-establish normality of thermo-regulation which, in turn, can help with many of the common skin problems of today.

4 Common skin problems today

Most common skin infections are well under control these days, largely as a result of good medical management and the use of antibiotics, antifungals and other medications. In their place, 'dermatitis' has risen to number one on the skin problems chart. As mentioned earlier, we use the term 'dermatitis' here generically, meaning any non-infectious inflammation of the skin, and thus indicating skin problems that may be lifestyle based or perpetuated. This can include a range of commonly known problems from simple rashes and persistent acne to eczema and psoriasis. Because our concern here is problems that are lifestyle dependent, they can often be modified by our own actions. It's these dermatitis-type problems to which we will limit our discussion.

Defining 'dermatitis'

Dermatitis, or inflammation ('itis') of the skin ('derma'), as a non-infectious, often lifestyle-based skin disorder, can be subdivided in many ways. Classifications can be based on morphology (appearance), location, cause (internal or external), histology (appearance under the microscope), age of onset, presence of secondary infection, or acuteness verses chronicity. Much has been written over the years in an attempt to differentiate one type of dermatitis from another.

An alternative approach is to consider many types of dermatitis to be reactions to skin *insult* of some form, either external or internal. To understand this, consider a personal insult: if you are insulted by someone, you can respond in a number of different ways; you can ignore it, laugh, cry, get angry, shout, threaten the insulter, attack or walk away. You might even do a number of these things at the same time. What you do depends largely on your personality and prior experiences. Your personality, in turn, is dependent on the interaction between nature and nurture. And while the former is difficult to manipulate, the latter can be significantly influenced by lifestyle change.

In a similar way, the skin reacts to insult, either external or organic, in a variety of ways. Such a reaction may show up as eczema, acne, psoriasis, urticaria, rashes, pimples or any number of other responses. The main thing is to understand that all forms of dermatitis are really just 'patterns of reaction' to insult in the skin. No one pattern is necessarily discrete or as clear cut as it may sound by the name which it is given. All need further description according to a number of factors—site, acuteness, age of onset, dryness or weepiness, presence of blisters (vesicles or bullae), weals, pain, itch, prickling and so on. But all are really just different reactions of the skin which come out in slightly different ways, depending on the interaction between the person and the type of insult.

Picture the skin, a large organ membrane, as possessing many abilities and functions, sitting between the inside of the body and a potentially hostile environment outside. As such, it is constantly buffeted from both sides, like the levees on a river bank during a flood, and the water is likely to break out anywhere and in a number of ways if the onslaught gets high enough. Given this picture, it's little wonder that factors such as the environment *outside*, and what is happening *inside*, are going to affect the skin. Preventing dermatitis must therefore involve keeping the skin in the best possible condition to resist any damage inflicted on it from either direction.

Over the last couple of decades, it has been shown that most of the responses which occur in the body to insult, injury or adverse situations are initiated and/or mediated by the production and circulation of *cytokines*, protein-like chemicals produced either in or around the distressed tissue. Cytokines are controlled by the immune system and may operate on their own or in association with antibodies. They may target just local tissues or they may affect distant organs, or both. They are attracted to cells which have specific cytokine receptor sites on their surfaces.

The above information should not be interpreted as a justification for the view that all dermatitis represents an allergic reaction of some type.

If a form of dermatitis does appear, it is vital to look for all possible causes and precipitants. When these have been identified (and in most cases there's a multiplicity of factors involved), steps can be taken to correct them and hence correct the problem itself. This can't always be done quickly, and sometimes it's not practical for a person to do it alone. As most people are aware, it generally takes time to get over a personal insult and for things to settle down—even after the appropriate apologies have been made. Where this happens in the skin, there might be value in using suppressants such as cortisone or other drugs to relieve symptoms, minimise the damage and prevent scarring, while the original condition responds to changes in habits, or lifestyle, or burns itself out—a bit like being soothed by a friend after an insult, until the memory of it goes away. Unlike the friend, though, all medical suppressants have side effects and complications which need to be delicately balanced against the benefits (see

Why do we sweat most from the head and face?

Most of the body's sweat glands are in a region from the nipple line to the top of the head. It's been proposed that this has developed through evolution as a means of dealing most effectively with body cooling. Air temperature is known to decrease logarithmically with the distance from the ground. Air speed also increases and this means sweat glands that are higher on the body will be more effective in cooling the body than those lower down. This has also been suggested as a reason why humans may have become upright rather than remaining on all fours like the apes from whom we have evolved.

Chapter 8). Such is the practice of dermatology—as indeed with most modern medicine.

Dr Eugene Farber of Stanford University in the United States talks about the 'iceberg' concept in skin disease. This considers the skin as one large, single organ, stretching from the scalp on the head to the soles of the feet. But just as we see only one-eighth of the iceberg above the surface (the remaining seven-eighths being below the water), when we see a rash on the skin we're only seeing the worst of the problem. Similar changes, albeit of less severity, are probably also taking place in the remainder of the skin. For this reason, when any part of the organ is out of order the whole skin should be cared for. It's our task here to determine just how this should be done and what you can do for yourself, without needing to call for the doctor. The first step is to look for some clues to the cause of the problem.

How location can be a clue to defining a skin problem

The location of a dermatitis can tell you a lot about its cause. Skin problems caused by sunlight, for instance, are usually limited to sun exposed areas of the body, as might be expected. Problems associated with overheating are usually more obvious in parts of the body with lots of sweat glands. For example, most sweating at night occurs in the 'heat sink' area from the nipple line to the scalp, where about 75 per cent of the body's sweat glands are resident, hence causing complications on the face and scalp. Sweating is also more prominent on the insides of the limbs than on the outsides, and on the lower part of the back and the groin. So a rash in these areas could well indicate sweat retention as a factor.

Some common types of skin problems where location can suggest the cause are those affecting the hands, feet and scalp. These parts of the body are associated with sweating (heat and stress) and thermo-regulation, and are areas which are commonly exposed to the environment and thus to environmental insult.

The hands and feet

The epidermis of the palms of the hands and the soles of the feet is much thicker than elsewhere. These areas also have no hair follicles or grease glands (*glabrous skin*), but they have a relatively large number of sweat glands compared to other parts of the body. They are both areas that are subject to insult of the physical and chemical type. Because of this, these two surfaces have become adapted to be resistant to such insult. Rarely do we find allergic contact dermatitis in these areas, for reasons we do not understand. It is unlikely to be due to the reduced ability for antigen presentation. Allergens and organisms on the skin surface need to be recognised and presented to the immune system before an appropriate response can occur. This is done by antigen *presenting cells* in the epidermis (Langehans cells and others) which are reduced in the palms and soles. Allergic reactions are much more common on the backs of the hands and tops of the feet. The picture is further complicated by the fact that patients with persisting palmar dermatitis are frequently found to react positively to patch testing to nickel and a few other common antigens, so the antigen must have been presented. Unfortunately, attempted complete removal of these antigens from contact with the skin—very difficult to do—including attempts to exclude nickel from the diet, have produced disappointing results. Nevertheless, the palms and soles are often involved in low-grade, non-infectious dermatitis caused by chronic irritation, both environmental and occupational. Because of the greater number of sweat glands under thermal and psychogenic influences, they are also affected by insults caused by overheating and stress. A dermatitis of the hands, for example, can develop in mothers who use Milton-type sterilisation solution for baby's bottles. This can continue even after the bottles have been put aside if the hands are being continually washed with detergent and/or if occlusive gloves are used in hot water or for long periods (see below).

There are similar problems with the feet because the skin can become dry from standing in the run-off from soaps and shampoos in the shower. Wearing modern shoes can make the problem worse because they can act like 'hot boxes' which continue the damaging effects of heating and drying. If a dermatitis starts on the feet, 'hot box' shoes can lead to a secondary infection with fungi, yeasts and low-grade bacteria and this may be called *tinea*, although the term is often used indiscriminately and, in reality, can include any one of a number of infections. Instead of dealing with this by applying expensive antifungal lotions and creams, it's probably best managed through prevention—by adequate moisturisation of the skin with simple applications such as Whitfield's Ointment aimed at 'waterproofing' the skin and keeping it acid so that fungi find it difficult to flourish. 'Treatments' often only serve to magnify the irritant condition and so insult the skin even further. Ventilation of the shoes can be very helpful (see Chapter 6).

The scalp

Another area where dermatitis often occurs is the scalp. Dandruff is common, and often this is just thought to be dead scalp tissue. Yet surprisingly there's not a lot known scientifically about dandruff. It is known that people with dandruff have a greater load on their scalp than normal of yeasts such as *pityrosporum*. But pityrosporum is normally present in the scalp anyway and this can multiply under certain conditions. Is this then the cause of dandruff, or the result? Irrespective, awareness of the increase in pityrosporum has led to the development of a vast array of commercial anti-dandruff treatments to kill off this overgrowth on the basis of it being the cause of the problem. As with other shampoos these products tend to dry out the scalp, and only serve to keep the dandruff temporarily off the shoulders if used daily. They should not be considered to provide a permanent solution.

An alternative view on dandruff is that sweat trapped in the dry skin of the scalp causes flaking of the scalp and the excessive growth of pityrosporum. As a result, the use of water soluble emollients—such as emulsifying ointment containing simple additives such as salicylic acid, tar and perhaps a little sulphur precipitate—when combined with a reduction in nocturnal over-heating have a better and longer lasting effect than traditional dandruff treatments.

Factitious ('person'-made) acne

Factitious acne, or facial dermatitis with acne-like spots, is another common modern skin problem which occurs particularly among young women with genetically dry skin. It is most common over the age of sixteen or seventeen (past puberty) in people who may have either had the odd pimple at puberty which then settled down, or have had no previous acne. Its onset coincides with the increased use of soaps, shampoos and time spent in airconditioned offices, centrally heated buildings and airconditioned cars. This type of acne is often itchy and is present on the central parts of the cheek, forehead and jaw line. It sometimes spreads to the shoulders and down the back and does not usually respond well to the accepted treatments for acne. Indeed, it's often made worse by drying or exfoliating agents, although it may respond temporarily to antibiotics and even to treatment with Roaccutane. However, even after this type of treatment it usually recurs within six to twelve months unless the causal factors are eliminated.

In people who suffer this condition, it's not unusual to find that they are overheating at night, often sleeping poorly, sometimes extending their hands and feet outside the bed covers during the night, waking up feeling tired, and having uncomfortable eyes (itchy, swollen, scaly, sleepy). When they get up in the morning their hair is often lank, greasy and dull. It can smell and feel 'damp' and the scalp can often be itchy and covered in dandruff. People with these problems have usually tried many 'cures', but mostly without success.

An enzyme system, the five reduction system, which can potentiate the effects of hormones (progesterone/testosterone) on the grease glands, can be increased by recurrent rubbing of the facial skin as occurs during overheating. Hence the cycle of overheating, rubbing and then washing, cleansing and drying can be the unseen perpetuator of the problem.

Factitious acne, so called because it is truly something with a lifestyle-based cause, has been found to respond well to cooling at night, avoidance of soaps and shampoos, the use of effective moisturisers (i.e. sorbolene and glycerine) all over the body, and more potent moisturisers (emulsifying ointment with 2–3 per cent salicylic acid—prescription required—mixed with a little water in the hands until creamy) on the upper body, face and scalp. This usually results in the rash settling down and the hair improving, as well as a general improvement in wellbeing and restedness after waking in the morning. The face may be irritable in the early stages, and this may be alleviated by the frequent application of 0.5 per cent hydrocortisone cream mixed with a little water in the first week or so and then slowly reduced.

Some before and after examples of this are shown in the photo section of this book.

Like all regimens involving lifestyle changes, this problem is not cured overnight. Full recovery often takes four to six months—a course of Roaccutane takes six months—and the procedures recommended in the next chapters are important for a full recovery.

Why does the skin in older people appear 'leathery'?

Leather is made from dried and treated animal skin. As with animals, drying and ageing of the skin in humans can result in the loss of its 'elastic' properties which enable it to 'snap' back into place after being extended. Instead of being in its natural, well ordered pattern, the elastic fibres of the aged skin become random and disrupted and give the appearance of 'deadness' and of animal 'leather'.

Non-location specific skin problems

There are exceptions to the locality theory of causality in dermatitis. Some forms of dermatitis have distinctive patterns of distribution which do not necessarily explain cause. Eczema, for example, is well known to be more common on the face and in the skin folds of the elbows and the knees, whereas psoriasis is more common on the outsides of the limbs, in the scalp and under and around the nails for no easily explainable reason. It has been suggested that the main recurring insult to the skin over the elbows and knees, where psoriasis is commonly found, could be the repeated stretching of the skin when the joints are flexed.

Other conditions such as *dermatitis herpetiformis* occur in areas subjected to pressure, such as the lower back, knees and elbows. Dermatitis associated with small blood vessels is more commonly found around the ankles and lower legs, slowly progressing in an upward direction. *Pityriasis rosea* occurs almost exclusively in areas protected from the sun and responds very well to gentle sunbaking. All of these things have to be considered if we want to find the cause of an eruption and treat it simply and effectively.

Genetic predisposition

Genetic predisposition is often an important factor in the background of many skin reactions including atopic eczema, psoriasis and even skin cancers, including some melanomas. Recognising the pieces of the jigsaw is important. However, genetic inheritance of more specifically defined abnormalities of the skin have been well documented over the centuries. The advent of modern scientific techniques has enabled us to start unravelling the various webs of mechanisms involved, but at this stage have not advanced therapy to very effective conclusions. We also can 'inherit' family practices, habits and traditions and, in contrast to genes, these can be changed.

Systemic/internal disorders

The presence of internal disease is often reflected in the skin, to the extent that the skin has been described as the body's 'distress flag'. Over the years, many texts and articles have been written on the topic of the dermatological signs of internal disease and there are now also several popular modern books relating skin disease to psychological problems. There's no doubt that the patterns and distribution of such signs of disease are signposts to be followed by a good practitioner in the investigation of the causes of skin problems. There's also little doubt that psychological problems such as stress, grief and bereavement can be reflected in skin problems. However, to blame psychological causes solely for all skin problems is dangerous and can obscure faulty lifestyle patterns or environmental determinants. This will be covered more in the following chapters.

Suppression of rashes

It has been said that 'a rash is a rash is a rash . . .' and if this is the case, any form of drug that suppresses a rash should work under all circumstances if a high enough dose is used. Unfortunately, this is not the case. Many rashes tend to recur unless the causes are detected and, wherever possible, eliminated. When the cause or the underlying precipitant, be it internal or environmental, cannot be identified, it may be necessary to use drugs to suppress the problem until the condition has 'burned itself out'. In this case, it is important to keep the dose of suppressant to a minimum, because all of these can carry their own complications which inevitably have to be dealt with (see Chapter 8). It is also vital that external causes, such as those discussed in the following chapters, be considered at least as contributing to the problem.

Skin cancer

While not strictly a form of dermatitis, skin cancer is a common form of skin problem in Australia with an environmental and lifestyle based cause. As most people are now aware, the most common forms of skin cancer are precipitated by damage to the skin due to sun exposure over an extended period. Even so, many other factors must be involved. Some people can suffer lots of sun damage but never seem to develop any detectable skin cancer. Others with a similar amount of damage might only develop recognisable signs of cancer at sites of additional injury, such as scars from chicken pox, vaccinations, burns or a sports injury. It is now generally accepted that sun damage resulting from cumulative exposure and sunburn in the first two decades of life seems to lay the foundation for the development of the common forms of skin cancer in later life.

People who are immuno-suppressed, either by disease (e.g. HIV) or drugs (e.g. transplant recipients), are also prone to skin cancer because of the reduced ability of their immune system to monitor early cancerous changes in the skin, and stimulate rejection. It is well known that some, probably many, skin cancers are adequately dealt with by the immune system without any outside help. Skin type also has an influence in the development of skin cancers and the most common types are discussed in the next chapter, along with other environmentally determined dermatitis.

Summary

The brief excursion we've made here into the most common skin problems of today has shown that there are many possible causes of modern non-infectious skin problems. Many of these, in turn, can be classified under the generic term 'dermatitis', although there are also other modern forms of environmental insult, such as skin cancer, which do not fit into this category. While some of these ailments have a genetic basis, and heredity can play a part in the development of others, it should be clear from our discussion of 'insult' to the skin that there are significant lifestyle and environmental factors which need to be discounted before any long-term treatment of many of these ailments is likely to be successful.

5 Environmental causes of skin problems

Once it is acknowledged that the environment and what we do to ourselves could be a source of many common skin problems, it becomes easy to see why these problems seem to be getting worse. In the past, humans have had to put up with the elements—sun, wind, cold, rain—with only clothes from animal skins and the occasional warm fire to keep their body temperatures within that narrow band that allows bodily organs to function satisfactorily. If the sun was too hot they kept out of it and retreated into the shade. Like many animals, they tended to rest in the shade during the day and travel or hunt during the cooler parts of the evening or night. If it was too cold they moved about more, covered themselves with whatever was available, used fires, pulled up an extra dog or two at night and generally sheltered from the weather.

Over the last 50 years, technology has provided us with a better understanding of insulation and with the means of achieving this through modern materials. We've also learned how to create artificial environments much more easily with the use of airconditioners and heaters. The problem with both of these, however, is that they tend to produce very dry air all year round, but even more so in winter when the air is already dry because of the cold. Heating cold, dry air results in an even greater lowering

Were the first humans dark skinned?

While it is impossible to answer this definitively, it seems quite probable that, as *Homo erectus* evolved in the equatorial regions of the earth and as darker skin provided protection against sunlight, evolution proceeded from dark to light. Fairer skinned people typically inhabit the higher latitudes where there is less sunlight and where fair skin is advantageous in trapping vitamin D from sunlight. Even today, Negroid peoples, particularly children, can develop vitamin D deficiencies living in latitudes even as relatively low as the United Kingdom because of the 'barrier' effect of dark skin against sunlight.

of humidity and drying of the skin. Humidification, which might help overcome this, is expensive and technologically difficult to achieve, particularly in environments such as aeroplanes. As early as 1972, a leading international dermatologist summed this up by claiming that:

> ... [the] man-made environment has become the most common cause of the incidence of dry skin and of the variety of cutaneous conditions resulting from this. Cleansing agents ... and rapid changes of temperature and humidity universally encountered either in overheating or airconditioning in homes, offices, airliners, and automobiles are among the modern, everyday environmental factors that contribute to the almost universal occurrence of dry skin.
>
> Chernosky, M.E., *Journal of the American Medical Association*, 1972

As we've seen, it is overheating and the dependence of individuals on artificial environments, rather than exercising the full range of their thermo-regulatory mechanisms, which has the potential for initiating many of the skin problems of today. The effects of heat and drying on skin, which is often inherently dry anyway, are among the most unrecognised causes of skin problems seen today. There are a number of environmental factors, both natural and unnatural, which can affect this.

With the great advances in technology there has developed a marked change in our ethos. Whereas in the past *survival* in the environment in which we functioned was our prime concern, in more modern times our thoughts have turned to ideas necessary to keep us *comfortable and beautiful*, using all the technology available. This exchange of goals has, in many ways, diverted us away from the environmental way of life. In the process we have often been deceived into thinking that comfort equates with safety.

Outdoors

Today, outdoor recreation is regarded, and no doubt is, a healthy past-time. But our attitude to exposure has changed. For the first time in history white-skinned people 'bake' in the sun in order to get the cosmetic effects of a suntan. Like people of all eras we seek comfort in warmth, unaware that the changes we have made to our indoor environments could result in them being a little too hot or a little too drying for a healthy skin.

In the outdoors, ultraviolet light from the sun is now accepted as a major cause of skin damage. Changes in the dermis, which reduce the ability of the epidermis to control its growth, are important as causative factors in skin cancer. But response to ultraviolet light is very variable. Dark skinned people are less likely to develop sun damage and subsequently develop skin cancers, but they are not

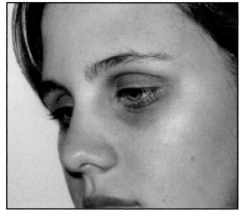

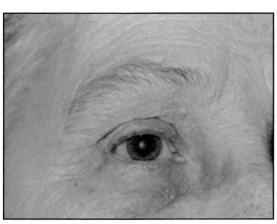

1 **Doona/duvet eye** Patient aged 29, had lived in Queensland all her life and used a doona all her life. Increased tissue formation above and below eyes, leading to hooding and baggy eyes, increased pigmentation. Itching settled with lifestyle changes. Pigment and bagginess will take a long time to settle. Note whiteheads on cheeks due to rubbing—leads to adult itchy acne.

2 **Rubbed eye** Overheating and dryness leads to rubbing at night producing whiteheads, blackheads, and causing enlargement of all minor excrescences.

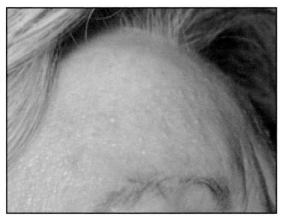

3 **Rubbed forehead** Dryness of skin and overheating at night leads to rubbing with the production of many whiteheads.

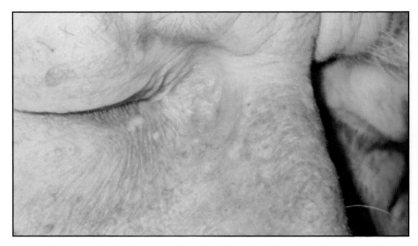

4a **Rubbed face due to dryness and overheating**   Leading to bagginess, whiteheads, blackheads and many enlarged warty spots.

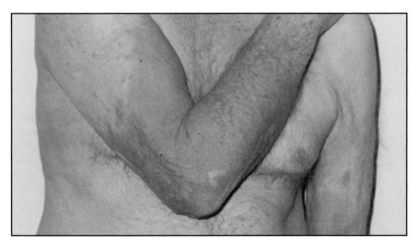

4b **Itchy dermatitis of arms (and legs)**   Due to dryness and overheating, leading to constant unconscious rubbing during the night.

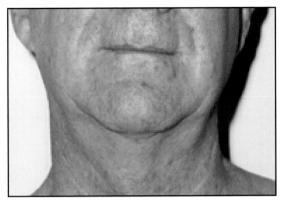

5a **Overheating** Constant red face with recurring pimples for twenty years or more. Regular use of antibiotics over this period helped only marginally.

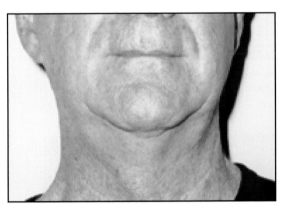

5b **One month later** Cooling, avoidance of soaps and shampoos, cessation of antibiotics and adequate moisturisation produced this dramatic result which has been maintained for over a year.

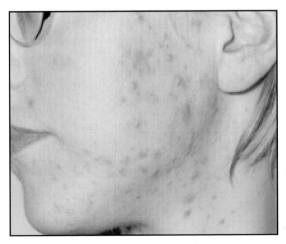

6 **Factitious acne** Aged 24, minimal previous acne. Backpacking in Australia for three months, sleeping in sleeping bag. Itchy facial adult acne caused by dryness, overheating and rubbing.

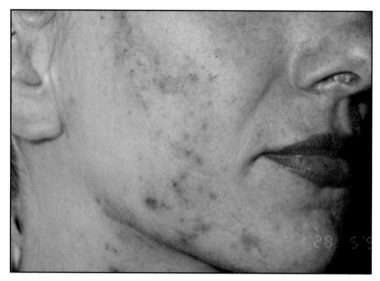

7a **Factitious acne**   Aged 23, no previous acne. No hormonal problems. Itchy adult acne after sleeping on heated waterbed with two doonas.

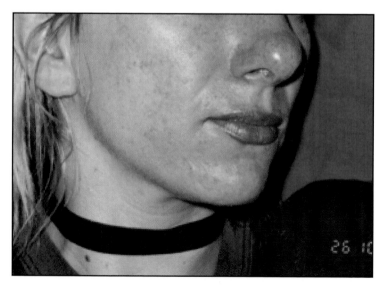

7b **Resolution in six months** with cooling, avoidance of soap and shampoo, adequate local moisturisation and simple local therapy.

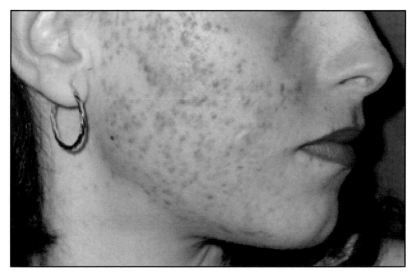

8a **Adult itchy acne**   Aged 23, lived in the tropics all her life. Commenced using a duvet/doona at 16 years. Acne-like eruption of face for five years, treated with antibiotics, hormones and three courses of Roaccutane.

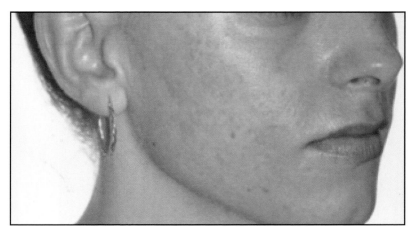

8b **Almost complete resolution** with minimal scarring after cooling down at night, no soap or shampoo, and adequate moisturisation with simple local therapy.

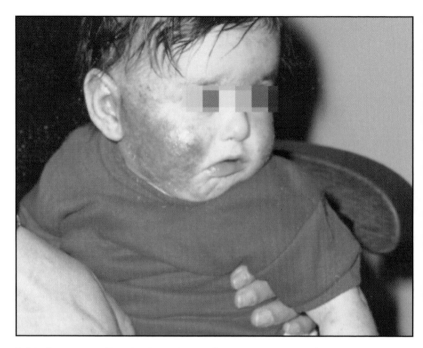

9 **Atopic eczema** Female, 4 months old. Severe eczema of the face, unresponsive to even potent local steroids. Little eczema elsewhere. Grossly overheated, 16 layers of clothing and bedding. Note sweaty hair. Mother afraid to reduce child's clothing, gradual deterioration of the eczema. Commenced refusing food and fluids. Admitted to intensive care because of heat exhaustion. Recovery slow.

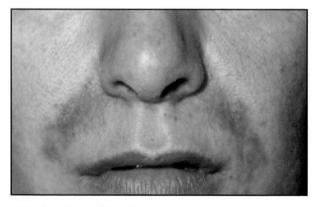

10 **Peri-oral dermatitis** Dry skin, overheating, anxiety, very itchy facial rash treated with strong steroids.

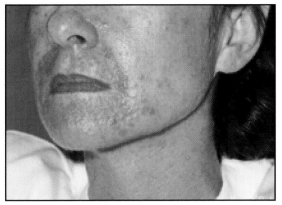

11a **Peri-oral and peri-orbital dermatitis** Patient aged 37 years, had lived in the tropics all her life. Hand eczema in the past, some degree of anxiety. Had used a doona/duvet for some years. Started with rash around mouth which gradually spread. Treatment with antibiotics, hormones and strong steroids with no improvement.

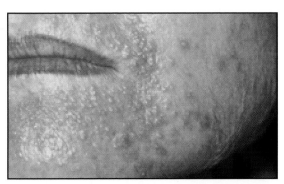

11b **Close up of typical peri-oral dermatitis**

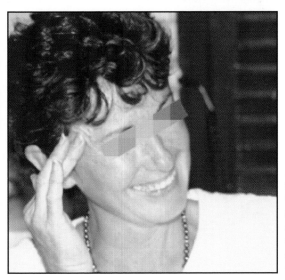

11c **Six months later,** marked improvement following cooling down at night, avoidance of soaps and shampoos, adequate moisturisation, a brief course of antibiotics and antihistamines.

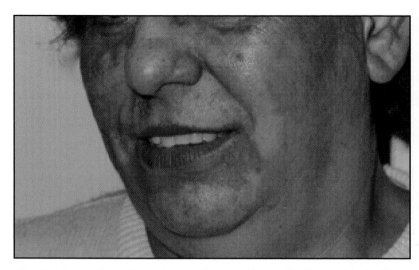

12a **Facial dermatitis with depigmentation** Dry skin, overheating at night leading to itching, rubbing and loss of pigment.

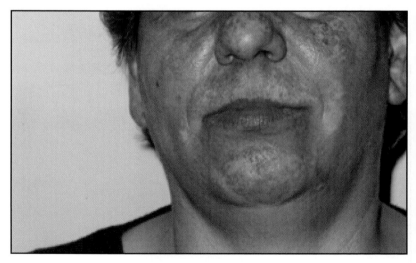

12b **Slow progress over six months** with keeping cool, no soaps or shampoos, adequate moisturisation and a very mild steroid cream. Gradual return of pigment is evident.

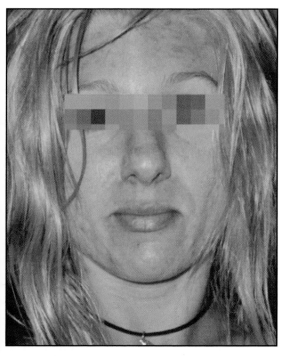

13a **Weathered hair**
Female 23 years of age,
sleeping on heated waterbed
with two doonas. Lank,
greasy hair, over-shampooed
and then bleached.

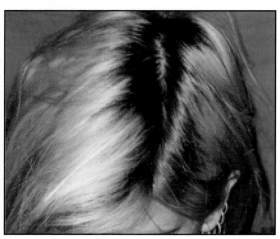

13b **Progress over six
months,** keeping cool,
using no soap or shampoo,
much better skin care.
Quality of hair much
improved.

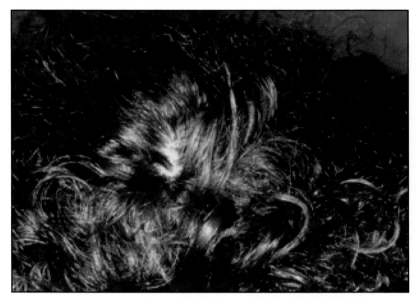

14 **Hair weathering** Hair damaged by overheating, over-shampooing and over-perming. Regrowth of 5cm good quality hair (black) at the rate of 1cm per month.

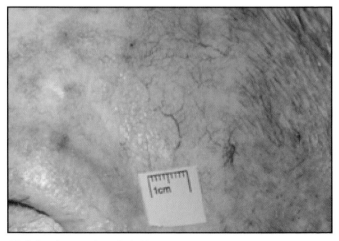

15 **Solar damage in a Celt** Note very thinned transparent epidermis, allowing visualisation of dermal papilli (small yellow lumps) and superficial blood vessels. This is a very severe example, with damage accumulated over many years.

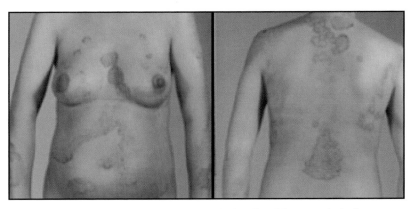

16a **Psoriasis** Female, late twenties, had suffered from psoriasis for many years and tried all the usual remedies. Sweating more during pregnancy, with psoriasis in areas of high sweating.

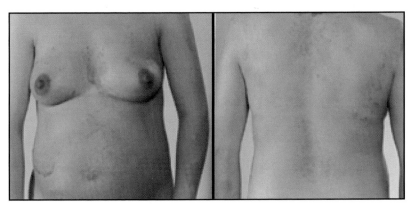

16b **Progress noted after six weeks** of keeping cool at night, avoiding soaps and shampoos and using a fairly heavy moisturiser all over the body at least once a day.

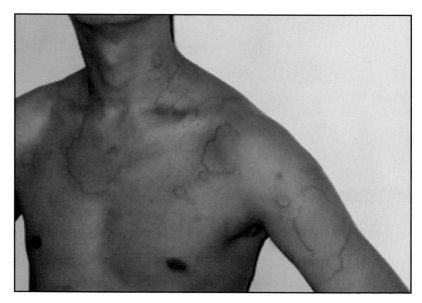

17 Urticaria Patient aged 36 years. Dry skin, overheating at night, recent distress over sudden death of a friend. Settled very quickly with keeping cool, avoiding soaps and shampoos, moisturising well and a short course of antihistamines.

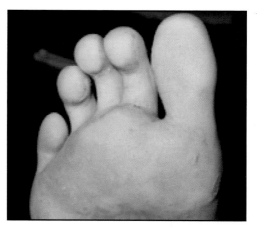

18 Pitted keratolysis (smelly feet). Male, late teens, dry skin, overheating at night and wearing 'hot box' shoes. Feet getting smellier every time they are washed with soap. Settled fairly rapidly with keeping cool at night, ventilating shoes, avoiding soap and shampoo, moisturising skin each day, and applying an acidified moisturiser to the feet twice daily.

Table 5.1: Skin classification based on reaction to sun exposure

Type	Skin reaction	Examples
I	Tans little or not at all, always burns easily and severely, then peels.	People most often with fair skin, blue eyes, freckles, white unexposed skin.
II	Usually burns easily and severely (painful burn); tans minimally and lightly.	People with fair skin, blue or hazel eyes, blonde or red hair, white unexposed skin.
III	Burns moderately, gains average tan.	Average Caucasian, white, unexposed skin.
IV	Burns minimally, tans easily and above average with each exposure.	People with light or brown skin, dark brown hair, dark eyes; unexposed skin is white or light brown (Asians, Hispanics, Mediterranean).
V	Rarely burns, tans easily and substantially.	Brown skinned persons; unexposed skin is brown (Indonesians, Hispanics, etc.).
VI	Tans profusely and never burns.	Persons with black skin.

totally immune. On the other hand, many fair skinned people who do not tan well and who have gross solar damage sometimes don't ever develop skin cancers.

It now seems obvious that some skin types are more easily damaged by sunlight than others. There is an accepted classification of skin based on its ability to tan, which has been in use for some years. This is shown in table 5.1 above.

Tips for avoiding skin problems from the sun

1. Only go into the sun when you have something sensible to do (this can include improving your state of mind), not just for the sake of being in the sun.

2. Try to limit sun exposure to the early morning and late afternoon periods, avoiding the hottest times of the day.

3. Wear reasonably protective clothing—baseball caps don't help very much (especially if they're worn backwards). Clothing with a high sun protective index is now available but, unfortunately, protection is only achieved by using close-knit materials, which can be very hot.

4. Use sun creams. Although there's a school of thought which questions the ability of these to prevent skin cancer, their use is still preferable to going without. On the other hand, there's little point in diligently applying a sun cream just to stay out in the sun longer.

5. Move around if you have to be out in the sun. If the hypothesis that sunburn is the major source of skin cancer in later life is correct, moving around should help to provide some protection. The child running around the beach all day develops an even overall tan while the child who falls asleep in the sun in its stroller will often get badly burned down one side of the body in a very short time.

Some forms of skin cancer do not seem to be associated with the direct effects of sunlight, but are more common in those people exposed to the sun. Melanoma, for example, can occur at any site where melanocytes can be found and the precipitating factors for this, other than sunlight and genetics, are not known. Melanomas can occur in places such as the mouth, vagina and rectum, where it is impossible to incriminate sunlight as a causative factor.

Even without developing skin cancer, sun damage, over time, tends to make the skin far less attractive with a leathery texture and much wrinkling and sagging. This is thought to be caused by the UVL (ultraviolet light) rays in sunlight which damage elastin and collagen fibres in the dermis, in the process now known as *solar elastosis*, recognised in the skin by a yellowish tinged lumpiness of the dermis as it appears through a thinned, semi-transparent epidermis. There's little or nothing that can be done about this, though some 'experts' promote rejuvenation with lasers and peeling, and some manufacturers promote the wonders of skin creams containing elastin and collagen. Retinoic acid was once advocated for rectifying the problem, but like many other miraculous remedies it now seems to be fading from use.

Despite our caution with regard to ultraviolet exposure, it must be remembered that some exposure to sunlight is important for a healthy life. Sunlight is essential for the formation of vitamin D in the body. It is also well known that sunlight produces a feeling of wellbeing in many people, and countries having long winters without much sunlight also have a high rate of a psychological ailment known as 'seasonal affective disorder' (SAD). In a country like Australia, adequate sunlight for health is available without having to venture outdoors for extended periods or to lie and 'bake' in the sun.

Sunglasses

Like the skin, the eyes require protection from UV light. Chronic exposure to sunlight can cause degenerative changes on the surface of the eye known as *pterygia*, and a degeneration under the cornea, in the lens. It is also suggested that the degenerative conditions of the retina occurring in the elderly, *macular degeneration*, is largely sun induced. Appropriate sunglasses can stop UV light reaching the eye, and it is obviously the sunglass lens which is important here. In a policy statement on the choice of sunglasses, the Australian College of Ophthalmologists has shown that the ability of the lens to protect the eye is not related to price. Standard plastic lenses transmit very little UV radiation and simple tinting and other treatment of the lenses can reduce this transmission to zero. The premium price paid for fashion sunglasses has little to do with eye protection, and a lot to do with the price paid for 'brand name' fashion.

A brimmed hat will reduce exposure to sunlight by roughly half, so this is the first and most direct line of defence for both the skin and the eyes. For maximum protection, sunglasses labelled as '100 per cent UV protective', or preferably '100 per cent absorbing below 400nm', should be chosen. To minimise entry of light around the frames, these should be of the wraparound style or with side 'blinkers'. It is not necessary to buy expensive sunglasses for full protection, and reasonable protection is afforded by many of the cheaper versions that can be bought at roadside service stations. Expensive 'name' brands of sunglasses (as worn and promoted by well-known international cricketers) may give more durability, comfort and 'style', but give little added protection for the price.

Cold

The advent of winter, while reducing the potential for skin cancers through sun exposure, brings its own problems. Cold air is usually dry, and this leads to a condition called *xerosis*, or 'dry skin', which in turn can lead to what is known as winter itch. This is most common in older people with good, or even excessive, hygiene, but who through ageing have an increasingly dry skin. Itching usually starts on the legs, arms and hips and is made more irritable by the use of deodorants and antiperspirants.

The dryness of the external air is often made worse by heating through artificial means and this can lead to a dermatitis with features of roughness, flaking, scaling, fissuring and apparent lack of moisture. The skin can become rough and harsh displaying redness, inflammation and irritated hair follicles, with many hairs broken off short. This condition was first described in 1874 but it was not until decades later that chapping of the skin due to dry air was offered as the explanation. A sudden drop in air temperature was thought to be the main precipitating factor, but in 1962 an American dermatologist reported the same problem in Texas arising from long periods of exposure to airconditioning, alternated with short exposures to a hot, humid outdoor environment. Winter itch, it seems, has achieved a longer life as a result of modern technology.

Indoors—at home

Probably more important than the natural environment and its effects on the skin are changes in our indoor environment. Advances in technology mean that we no longer have to put up with discomfort—we can stay warm, in fact hot, for 24 hours of the day if we like. This is reflected in housing in the western world, which has undergone dramatic changes in the past few decades. There is widespread use of central heating and cooling, both of which reduce relative humidity in buildings, both workplace and home. Double glazing is now widespread and this adds to the central heating or cooling effects to reduce the moisture content of the air. Heating and cooling even in the modern car has eliminated the effects of the natural environment. As a result, the body's thermo-regulatory system becomes inefficient and ineffective in managing even small changes in temperature. In the meantime our addiction to warmth and dryness means the skin dries out, loses its moderating potential and becomes more vulnerable to the range of insults which can result in dermatitis.

Bedding

One of the biggest and most unrecognised potential skin problems in the indoor environment is modern bedding. The continental quilt (duvet, doona, etc.), as the name implies, was initially Europe's answer to freezing, blizzardy, snow-filled winter nights. More recently they've been promoted throughout the western world, including Australia.

Originally, doonas were stuffed with feathers or wool, but now these fillings are usually replaced with synthetic material which is light to use and easily kept tidy.

There are no standards for the thermal insulation capacity of blankets, quilts, doonas or duvets in Australia. In the United Kingdom, standards are established by the British Textile Technical Research Group (BTTRG) at Shirley Towers. They advocate a unit of Thermal Insulation Capacity which they call a TOG rating. Garments and bedding are now labelled according to their TOG rating. Table 5.2 shows the TOG rating of various items of clothing and bedding as determined by the BTTRG.

Additional Australian estimates of the TOG value of various items shown in table 5.3 have been made by Dr Don Hutton of the Physics Department at Monash University in Melbourne. These show some differences from the British figures because of possible differences in material and the difficulty in accurate measurements of this kind. These figures are old and no more recent ones are to hand. Bedding manufacturers have also modified their products in the meantime, but the habit of overheating at night persists in some households.

Table 5.2: Typical thermal resistance (TOG) values

Covering	TOG value
Shirting—cotton	0.1
Underwear	0.2–0.4
Thermal underwear	0.4–0.8
Suiting	1.0
Sweaters/jumpers	1.0
Blankets	1–2
Continental quilt (doona)	10

Table 5.3: Australian measures of thermal resistance

Covering	TOG value	Covering	TOG value
Open weave singlet	0.2	Thermal singlet	0.4
Cotton shirt	0.7	Woollen shirt	0.9
Woollen jumper	1.0	Fleece jacket	1.5
Light pyjamas/nightie	0.5	Heavy pyjamas/nightie	1.0
Sheet	0.5	Blanket	1–2
Thin doona	2.5–4.0	Thick doona	6–10

In their literature, the BTTRG suggest that a 9 TOG doona should keep a person comfortably warm in bed when the room temperature is 5°C. It's estimated that the minimum bedroom temperature in unheated bedrooms in Sydney in winter, in a wooden house with a window partially open, rarely falls below 10°C. In Melbourne, and further south in Tasmania and in the alpine country, bedroom temperatures fall further than this, but are much less than would be experienced outside. Most modern houses are well insulated and there is residual heat left over from the day, reducing the need for heavy bedding.

As can be seen from table 5.2, the average doona has been found to be equivalent in thermal insulation capacity to 9–10 TOGS, while a wool or cotton blanket was found to equal 1–2 TOGS. Hence a doona is equivalent in insulation to five or six blankets. The biggest disadvantage of a doona, however, is that this cannot be discarded in sections (peeled off) as blankets can be during the night. The body heats slowly, almost imperceptibly. And while there's always the tendency to 'jump start' this by bounding into a cosy, pre-warmed bed, the heating effect can often 'overshoot'. You're probably well into a deep sleep by the time your body temperature rises significantly. If it keeps rising, you start to sweat. You might throw off the whole doona to try to compensate for this, but because the body cools much quicker than it heats (within 3 to 4 minutes), it's not long before you're cold and have to pull the doona back into place.

Sweating under a heavy cover is not an effective way to control body temperature, as can be seen in diagram 5.1. The doona doesn't allow the sweat to evaporate off the skin, and so natural cooling doesn't occur. Unless a leg or an arm is stuck out from under as a temporary 'thermostat', the only part of the body where heat loss can occur is that part exposed to the air, usually the head and neck. Such bouts of sweating occur during periods of light sleep, mostly at about 2 am, and are often associated with facial rubbing and head scratching. These can cause problems like those shown in the photo section of the book.

Problems associated with overheating at night

Poor sleep

Sleep quality decreases with higher body temperatures. Bed temperatures above about 32°C reduce rapid eye movement (REM) sleep, which is very important for quality sleep. Without it, you can feel tired and washed out during the day—as if you have a hangover but haven't been drinking. The effect can be reduced in

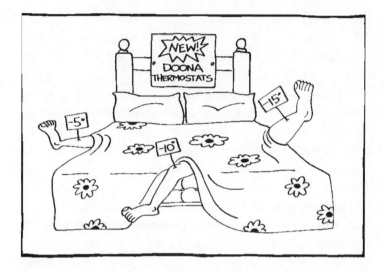

the overheated bed by sticking the hands or feet out from under the doona, or throwing the bedding off during the night, but this is only a short-term solution because cold is quickly felt and the extreme warmth of the doona becomes more attractive until overheating again builds up slowly, hence perpetuating the cycle.

The study of alterations in brain waves during different sleep stages has shown that people who are too hot at night spend more time in light sleep and less time in deep sleep than is considered normal for their age and sex. Often this is not recognised, although a sleeping partner may be aware of it from the tossing and turning that occurs, particularly in the early hours of the morning. Older people who may have taken sleeping tablets to overcome their insomnia, frequently caused by overheating, often fail to cool off during the night and can often wake with itchy legs and widespread and resistant lower leg dermatitis as a result. Leg cramps can also be associated with being too hot.

'Doona eyes'

'Doona eyes' is a term given to the darkening of skin around the eyes as seen in the photo section. This can result from increased tissue formation in the upper eyelid, spreading around the eyes and leading to hooding and bagginess, with increased folding of the upper lid. Sufferers often complain of itchiness, flaking, swelling of the eyelids and mucus (or 'sleep') in the eyes on waking. The problem is often put down to stress or tiredness, but is more directly attributable to the poor sleep associated with overheating. During the night the sensation of discomfort around the eyes caused by sweating about the head can cause excessive rubbing and this can exacerbate the problem by causing conjunctival irritation and even sub-conjunctival haemorrhage. Such changes take years to regress.

After going to bed under a doona, body temperature will rise slowly over the next two to three hours while warm air circulates under the covers. Overheating may not be felt until you have been asleep for two to three hours. Sweat produced in the scalp combines with the grease there to make a thick, tacky emulsion which can only be removed by the regular use of very strong detergent shampoo, which can then dry and damage the hair and skin.

Facial dermatitis

If facial rubbing during the night extends beyond the limits of the eye many other skin changes become noticeable, including increasing redness, thickening and some scaling amounting to a low-grade dermatitis. This may respond initially to local application of steroid creams, but will probably return when these applications are ceased if the underlying causes are not dealt with. It is often treated as *rosacea*, responding poorly and only partially.

Repeated rubbing causes small excrescences or lumps around the eyes and on the face to enlarge and multiply. It also causes

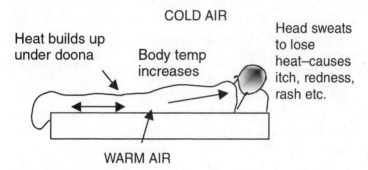

Diagram 5.1 How doonas can cause skin problems

the formation of comedones (blackheads and whiteheads) which present on the forehead, cheeks and chin. These are the basis of adult itchy acne or factitious acne seen on the faces of many females who are well past puberty and have no apparent hormonal problems to account for their acne. (This is sometimes colloquially called 'checkout chick's face'.) They don't respond to the usual forms of therapy such as antibiotics, cleansers, exfoliants or lotions containing alcohol and propylene glycol. However, they do respond, in a matter of a few months, to better environmental care and lifestyle change (about the same time as it takes for a course of Roaccutane to work but the result is more sustained).

Perioral dermatitis

In the late 1960s and early 1970s, a skin condition described as *perioral dermatitis*, which had not previously been described, came to the notice of dermatologists (see photo section). Its distribution seemed to be confined to the western world, and its signs and symptoms were so well defined that it could not be thought of as anything but a single entity. No one was able initially to explain why it occurred. Treating the condition was difficult in the early stages, although it did seem to respond well to steroid creams (especially the new ones described as 'fluorinated'). Unfortunately, it was soon found that the remarkable improvement produced by the steroids was followed by a severe rebound of both the rash and the symptoms within ten to fourteen days of ceasing the application. The appearance of this new condition, with hindsight, appears to have coincided with the renewed popularity of the doona and the release onto the market of the stronger fluorinated steroid creams. Original investigations and comments by Dr I. Sneddon in the United Kingdom proved very helpful with regard to its treatment.

Grover's disease

This is not related to watching too much *Sesame Street*, but was named after the New York dermatologist who discovered it in the 1970s. The disease is distinguished by itchy red lumps occurring on the upper chest of middle-aged men, most of whom seemed to spend much of their time in New York offices followed by a two to three week holiday lying in the sun in places such as Florida. For this reason the problem was thought to be related to sunlight. It was itchy and annoying, especially in bed at night. Some patients appeared to respond to the stronger steroid creams, but others did not. Specimens examined under the microscope showed a variety of patterns, but all contained cells which had been split off from their neighbours, known as *acantholytic cells*. Hence the condition became known as *acantholytic dermatosis*.

It was soon realised that sweat entrapment was a major factor in the cause of this ailment, and that this was more likely to be due to overheating rather than to sunlight. The variation in microscopic appearance around the acantholytic cells supports the notion of *reactive dermatitis,* which clearly labels it as a response to some external cause. Occasionally this condition assumes a chronic phase resembling a widespread itchy dermatitis that does not resolve, even with high doses of cortisone, but will settle down with the addition of retinoids provided the usual precautions are taken to adequately moisturise the skin and avoid overheating at night.

Facial excrescences

Repeated nocturnal rubbing tends to cause any small abnormal growths (irregularities) around the eyes or on the face and forehead to enlarge and multiply. Many so-called solar keratoses (sun spots) can react in this way. They are usually treated by freezing, but if overdone this may leave a white spot on the skin. A more effective treatment with less damage than liquid nitrogen generally results in the problem settling down in a short time, provided the appropriate lifestyle changes, such as adequate moisturising and a decrease in nocturnal overheating, are instituted. It is now realised that less than 1 in 1000 solar keratoses proceed to full cancer.

Atopic eczema and acne

Atopic eczema is known to frequently first appear on the faces of infants at about the age of six months. This is often seen in the absence of eczema elsewhere on the body and is found in many children who are grossly over-clothed, with hair matted with perspiration and face and hands being the only exposed areas of the body for effective heat loss (see the photo section). The facial sweating is accompanied by frequent facial rubbing.

Routine pubertal acne, which appears to be getting worse in modern society, is often also associated with the use of drying medications and overheating at night. Changing lifestyle, particularly those factors leading to overheating at night, can go a long way, if not all the way, to dealing with the problem. Adequate moisturising is also essential.

Hair and scalp problems

Although it is difficult to quantify sweat loss through the head at night because of differences in hairstyle and length, it is obvious that people who overheat at night do a good deal of sweating through the head.

Lank, greasy, uncomfortable hair in the morning is a common complaint associated with such sweating (it's often thought to be just a 'bad hair day') and this can be made worse by what you might do to correct it. Jumping into a shower, scrubbing the face with soap and shampooing the hair to get rid of that 'dead' feeling could be counterproductive. Because soaps and shampoos are like detergents (see Chapter 7) they cleanse the skin and hair of all their natural oils and actually make them drier, more itchy and more prone to skin problems. (Changes in hair after introducing cooling procedures are shown in the photo section.) Many males have attempted to eliminate the problem these days by simply shaving their heads.

Other signs

Overheating during sleep can lead to breathing through an open mouth, like a dog panting over its extended tongue. This can cause a drying up and irritation of the throat and soft palate leading to snoring, a problem which is even worse in the overweight because of the occlusion of the pharynx, or windpipe, by an enlarged tongue. Overheating of this type can also cause drying of the nasal passages, giving rise to morning sneezing and a runny nose on waking, which is often misinterpreted as a cold or viral infection. Constant mouth breathing can dry the lower lip, initiating frequent lip-licking and the development of *salivary cheilitis* (inflammation of the lip).

Existing skin conditions can also be aggravated by being too hot at night. This might manifest as a dry itch of the shoulders and upper back, areas of hypo-pigmentation (*pityriasis alba*), worsening of white spot disease (*tinea versicolor*), and even vesicular (weeping) eruptions on the palms of the hands and soles of the feet (*pompholyx*). Other problems such as hives can result from a combination of dryness, overheating and psychological stress (see the photo section).

The problems of heat build-up at night

The slow build-up of heat in the body means that climbing into an already overheated bed, such as with an electric blanket, could be a particular problem, especially if the heat is not reduced before you go to sleep. A slight amount of discomfort in the early stages of warming might be a safeguard against overheating later in the night. An electric blanket with a doona is a recipe for skin problems.

Replacing a doona with blankets, especially in heated houses, can help resolve many skin problems, including what is often labelled as scalp psoriasis, 'zits' or acne, redness and itchiness of the face and head, and lank, dry and lifeless hair. Woollen and cotton blankets are preferable to acrylic, mohair or angora blankets which, although lighter, retain more heat during the night. Table 5.4 gives a rough guide used in clinical practice for the optimal number of blankets to use at night, based on the minimum bedroom temperature (MBRT) as estimated with no artificial heating and with a window slightly open.

Bed clothing

Clothing in bed serves a number of functions. Obviously, it can help keep us warm, particularly in the early stages of the night before

Table 5.4: Guide to optimal bedding based on room temperature

MBRT (4 am–5 am)	Blankets (cotton/wool)
20°C and above	1 cotton sheet
16°C	1–2 cotton sheets
13°C	1 cotton sheet and 1 blanket
11°C	2 blankets
9°C	3 blankets
7°C and below	4 blankets

body temperature starts to rise. But perhaps the most important function is the stabilisation of the thin layer of air around and close to the skin. Sleeping nude can cause irritations to the skin by the disruption of this layer of air each time we turn over. Thick, heavy clothing on the other hand, such as a tracksuit with bedsocks, will soon cause overheating and the sweating known to cause skin problems. A rational middle solution is to wear thin, comfortable bed clothes all through the year to preserve the layer of air next to the skin. Variations in bedding, such as a number of sheets and/ or blankets which can be shed individually through the night, can help cope with any external temperature changes. Many of these problems settle down after an initial period of discomfort which occurs during the period or retaining of the thermo-regulatory mechanisms (TRM). It is usually not helpful to try to cover this period by resorting to taking sleeping tablets for more than a couple of nights maximum. No gain without pain.

The main sites for controlling heat loss apart from sweating are the extremities of the body, the hands and feet. If these are covered at night, such as with bed socks, the ability of the body to lose heat is compromised and an even greater degree of overheating can occur. For this reason bed socks are not recommended. On the other hand, cold feet can be a problem for people with TRM who may find it

Tips for avoiding overheating at night

1. Don't overheat the bed before getting in.
2. Accept that it is not necessary to have warm feet on getting into bed.
3. If necessary, warm the feet with a towel heated in the microwave.
4. Use blankets and sheets instead of a doona.
5. Peel off blankets progressively as the body heats up.
6. Wear light bed clothing all year round.

difficult to get off to sleep without added heating. However, continuing to use these devices could be counterproductive. Cold feet can best be dealt with by warming a small towel in a microwave with a small glass of water for two to three minutes and placing it under the feet at the end of the bed. This will warm the feet enough to get off to sleep, and then rapidly cool down when it's no longer necessary. This approach is very effective with children and much safer than a hot water bottle, particularly for those who may be diabetic, or potentially diabetic, and who may have lost sensation in the extremities.

Indoors—at work

The modern work environment can also be a cause of skin troubles. Airconditioning systems in the office extract water vapour from the air before it is circulated, thereby creating a 'hostile' environment for the skin. 'Sick building syndrome' has recently been used to describe a collection of symptoms, including respiratory problems and dried out skin, that afflict office workers. This has variously been ascribed to circulating microbes in the airconditioning, but it's more likely to be a result of the airconditioning itself. In addition, there's a suggestion from some researchers that 'red faces' attributed to working with VDUs might result, at least in part, from dryness and overheating in offices.

Unlike at home, it's often difficult to change the work environment. Some changes which may be helpful include having a few bowls of water strategically placed around the office and opening windows where possible. Try to take regular breaks outside the office, avoiding the cigarette smokers. Moisturiser applied to the skin daily, as often as possible (a little and often), can help prevent drying. It's far better to apply a little of this frequently than a lot occasionally.

'Screen dermatitis' is the name given to an increasingly common skin problem associated with electrical equipment, and particularly video display terminals. General symptoms can include dizziness, tiredness and headache, and effects on the skin can be *erythema* (redness), heat sensation, swelling and pain similar to that suffered from sunburn. The effect may simply be due to dryness of the office environment, giving rise to irritation of the skin and consequent facial rubbing. In any case, the obvious treatment is prevention, by not being exposed. However, milder symptoms may be reduced by maintaining air moisture, such as through a constant bowl of water on the desk, and by regularly waterproofing the skin through the use of a moisturiser.

Stressful situations, both at work and in domestic and social situations, can also lead to problems. The relationship between stress and the skin is well noted. This relationship is not surprising since the skin is an organ of communication, often referred to as the body's 'distress flag'. In the early stages of development of the foetus, some cells form the neural crest which goes on to form the frontal lobes of the brain, the pigment cells of the skin

Tips for avoiding skin problems from work

1. Keep a bowl of water full and handy to your desk.
2. Take regular breaks outside.
3. If possible, open windows and allow external air to circulate.
4. Have techniques available for dealing with stressful situations.
5. Try to maintain a normal body weight by being active around the office.
6. Take regular breaks from VDUs.
7. Keep a moisturising cream in the office and use regularly.

(melanocytes) and the factory cells of the skin (mast cells), which produce many chemical messengers such as histamine. It is not surprising, therefore, that these three different types of cells, which have a common ancestry, should share many common chemical mediators and messengers and, as a consequence, relate to each other in certain circumstances. If a person is stressed by problems at home or at work, it is understandable that his or her skin may react adversely. It is also understandable that some drugs discovered in the search for antihistamines and antidepressants should be related. The interaction between stress and the environment is also important, so alleviating stress can often be an aid to improved skin.

The 'travelling skin'

Increasing prosperity has meant an increase in world travel. But the international traveller is certainly not free from the ravages of the man-made environment. Long-haul flights mean sitting for hours in planes where the relative humidity can be very low. This tends

Tips for avoiding skin problems while travelling

1. Pack a moisturiser and use often in planes or airconditioned vehicles.
2. Switch off the airconditioner in your hotel.
3. Open the windows if possible in a hotel or fill the bath full of water.
4. Use a fine spray mist in the car if the windows can't be opened.
5. Avoid airconditioners and heaters where feasible.
6. Try to find a hotel that supplies blankets rather than doonas.
7. Try to take regular breaks in the outdoors.

to dry out the skin and mucous membranes and helps explain that washed out, tired look when you arrive at your destination.

Even the local traveller has problems these days. Cars, which used to have side windows to allow some air in for cooling while the main window was closed, have now changed. In their place is the car aircon for summer or the heater for winter, both of which dry out the interior of the car and cocoon it from the natural atmosphere. Over a long trip this can dry you out like a prune and leave you feeling irritable and exhausted when you arrive at your destination. One way of rectifying this is to spray a fine mist of water into the air every now and then from a spray bottle left in the car over long journeys, particularly those in winter when the air is drier.

If you're travelling you might book into a hotel or motel when you arrive, most of which have airconditioning, drying out the inside atmosphere. If, as in many of the larger hotel chains, the windows can't be opened, you're caught in a veritable drying pit—even though it might be cool! Propping open the bathroom door and keeping the bathtub full of water throughout your stay can go some way towards relieving the problem. Also, regular use of a skin moisturiser both during a flight and on the ground can provide relief from the excessive dryness that leads to skin problems.

6 Technology and the skin

Major changes in living environments for humans over the past century have been caused and accompanied by big advances in technology. And while there's no doubt that this has improved the living conditions of the human race, it also has a downside. This is not to take a Luddite approach to technology. It is merely to point out that there is a flipside to every coin and that the flipside in this case can be reflected in problems in the human skin.

Technology, obesity and skin problems

After an evolutionary history of leanness, human beings, at least in advanced societies, are now fat, very fat. Around 67 per cent of men and 55 per cent of women in Australia in 2000 were classified as overweight or obese. What does this have to do with skin, you might say (apart from requiring more of it)? Surprisingly, a lot. As you can see by now, the general thesis of this book is that lifestyle, and particularly overheating, can cause skin problems. Fat is one of the body's great insulators. It holds in heat and keeps out cold. Where sweating occurs, such as under mounds of flesh (around the abdominal apron in fat men, or under the breasts of fat women), waterlogging and dermatitis can result. Hence, if dealing with the problem means dealing with the cause, the causes of obesity, and the reason it's so common, need to be understood.

It's no secret how we get fat. It comes from an imbalance of too much energy (food and drink) taken in, with too little energy (movement) expended. It's not coincidental, therefore, that advances in technology can cause obesity. Obesity in turn can cause skin (and other) problems. To reduce obesity, a balanced food intake needs to be considered (not a diet in the sense of severely restricting food), but perhaps more importantly an increase in physical activity or movement throughout the day. This could be through planned actions, such as going for a walk, riding a bike or playing sport, but just as importantly it could be through using the stairs instead of the escalator, not using the remote control on the TV or garage door, or walking across the office floor to talk to a workmate rather than sending an e-mail.

Obesity is one of the unrecognised associates of skin problems. *Intertrigo* is the name given to a red, irritable, inflammatory condition which occurs in skin folds, and is more common in obese people.

Dermatitis can occur on any part of the foot; the localisation seems to depend on the precipitating factors. These can include drying, waterlogging, primary irritation, allergic reactions, physical stresses and footwear trauma. Pedal skin tends to dry out because of exposure to the air, the effects of soaps, detergents and shampoos etc. Such skin is then very vulnerable to waterlogging by sweat resulting from the wearing of unsuitable ('hot box') shoes. When this occurs, the skin is more vulnerable to in-shoe trauma and it becomes alkaline which enables yeasts, fungi and certain types of bacteria to flourish on the surface and infect it. Synthetic and rubber footwear are more likely to cause the waterlogging, and thongs to cause drying out. Thongs, especially when the heel extends over the back of the sole, are the most common cause of heel fissuring.

The soles are rarely involved in allergic reactions, whereas the upper surface is often involved, as with the hand. Obesity plays a large part in this.

The use of old-fashioned terms such as 'athletes foot' and 'trench foot' tends to confuse the picture. Even the term tinea pedis has lost its significance these days because, strictly speaking, it refers to pure, uncomplicated fungal infections. Foot dermatitis is a far more realistic term to use.

Pitted keratolysis is a term used to describe a very smelly, frustrating dermatitis of the soles and toe webs caused by a mixture of all the above, which gets smellier the more it is washed with soap, detergents, antiseptics etc. It settles down very quickly once attention is paid to all the environmental factors. Heat and sweating should be dealt with. Soaps and shampoos should not be used. The feet may be washed with moisturising cream and then liberally moisturised with a mixture of Whitfield's ointment and water three to four times daily.

Skin tags are also more common in the obese. *Acanthosis nigrocans*, a dark, velvety folded skin change which occurs under the arms and in the groin, is also associated with obesity and the likelihood of developing diabetes.

Ironically, excess body fat is not only responsible for skin problems because of heat, but excess heat can be a cause of excess body fat. The body's metabolism is known to be slowed by exposure to constant heat. Metabolism, in turn, is the body's 'engine' and, like any engine, the higher this is turned up the more energy it uses. Resting metabolism accounts for about 70 per cent of our total daily energy expenditure. If this is decreased, even by 10 per cent, it can account for over 400 kilojoules of energy per day being conserved. As 1 kilogram of fat is the equivalent of about 32,000 kilojoules, this means, in theory at least, that about 4.5 kilograms

How your doona could be making you fat

Increases in body temperature can lead to a decrease in metabolic rate. This is because the body does not have to 'work' to produce energy for heat maintenance (as it does in the cold, through shivering). Use of a heavy doona at night prevents heat loss from all over the body and only allows it through that part of the body exposed to the air (usually the head, or an arm or leg if it is stuck out during the night—see next chapter). This increases total body temperature and hence has the potential of lowering metabolic rate. A lower metabolism leads to less energy use and therefore the greater potential storage of fat—meaning your doona could be making you fat!

a year could easily be gained (all else being equal) by slowing down metabolism this much. Hot weather, constant exposure to warm air and sleeping in overheated conditions such as under a doona can have this effect. So while the environment could be affecting your skin directly, it could also be doing so indirectly through increasing body fat.

Clothing

Synthetic fibres are now incorporated into much modern clothing and bedding. They're cheaper than natural fibres, wear better, are lighter, less bulky and are often better insulators. Over 5 to 10 per cent of these fibres, even when mixed with natural fibres, tend to cause a build-up of heat. Many people feel uncomfortable in clothing made from synthetic fibres.

Exercise clothing

Sport or exercise can be a particular problem for the skin, because sweating is usually a necessary by-product of physical exertion. The function of sweat, of course, is cooling. But for sweat to be effective in cooling, it has to be evaporated off the skin. If the type of clothing doesn't allow this, skin problems can result. Cyclists who wear full-length lycra suits are especially prone to these problems. Joggers, who think that running in a heavy tracksuit with gloves and cap is going to help them 'sweat weight off', are equally deluded. While they may lose 'weight', this is only water through sweat, not fat, and it will quickly return with rehydrating after exercising. In the meantime, there's a build-up of heat on the skin that is not dissipated and is likely to cause itchiness and irritation; this is then made worse by washing and scrubbing to get rid of the itch. The same applies to many of the rubber/synthetic suits sold with a view to encouraging weight loss. Not only are these ineffective in 'spot reduction' as they are often advertised, but can be potentially irritating to the skin.

Synthetics such as nylon, often used as inserts in swimwear, can become abrasive once damp. The use of such clothing when jogging or exercising frequently causes traumatic dermatitis of the groin and other areas. Exercise clothing is best derived from natural fibres with the extremities (arms and legs) kept bare and a bare midriff. It should also be as loose as possible so as not to cause frictional damage.

Children's wear

Avoiding synthetic clothing might be sound advice for adults, but what about children who have their choices made by adults? Parents universally feel that their offspring are more vulnerable to the effects of climate than adults. They fail to understand that heat loss from the hands and feet is important for the control of body temperature and that covering these with gloves, bootees and bonnets in a way that would suit the Inuit of Alaska can be potentially damaging to the child's skin. In a normally mild climate such as Australia's, this just helps to upset the normal thermo-regulatory mechanisms and cause greater potential problems later in life. It also compromises the child in its attempt to mature its TRM. The head, and more specifically the face, becomes the main site for heat loss from the over-clothed child. This is made even worse if an over-clothed child's head is covered, and may rapidly complicate an already serious situation. Atopic eczema in infants frequently presents on the cheeks and chin between the ages of six and twelve months. Sweating leads to itching, which leads to rubbing and scratching

It's quite possible that much bad-tempered behaviour in children results from over-clothing. In a survey conducted in the United Kingdom in 1986, it was found that of 200 babies visited by health visitors in their homes, 5 per cent were visibly sweating and at least one-third were considered to be over-clothed. The amount of clothing worn bore little or no relationship to the temperature inside the house, but in many cases depended on an assessment of the weather outdoors viewed by the parent or guardian through the double-glazed windows!! Possible relationships between overheating and sleep disorders and psychological and behavioural disorders in children are also currently under investigation.

Many years' experience in practice by HM have taught a number of lessons. Screaming, angry children dragged into the consulting room by distraught parents were often over-clothed. The simple way of dealing with this is to say that one needs to examine ALL of the child's skin and so ALL of the clothing should be removed at

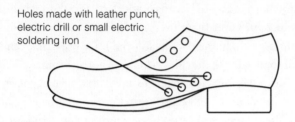

Holes made with leather punch, electric drill or small electric soldering iron

Diagram 6.1 Footwear ventilation

once. Within five minutes of this being done, the children were like 'lambs in the field'.

Footwear

Modern footwear can also present problems for the skin. Contemporary shoes, as a result of modern manufacturing techniques, have become 'hot boxes' from which heat has difficulty in escaping. The uppers are often made of synthetic material or, if made from leather, are sprayed with 'anti-scuff' applications in order to reduce the need for polishing. As a result, air is unable to circulate and the inside of the shoe is turned into a kind of steam bath, which provides an ideal environment for all forms of skin problems, including tinia pedis and pitted keratolysis.

This can be overcome by ventilating the shoes, by making a few small holes in the upper, in the area of the instep approximately 1 cm above the welt. This allows air to flow through the instep on each step like a form of bellows and can reduce the internal temperature of the shoe by up to 3°C. Surprisingly, ventilated shoes do not give rise to wet feet when it rains.

Foot problems are a particular issue in people with diabetes. This is because of the secondary complications that occur due to small blood vessel and sensory nerve damage; this can accentuate the damage caused by minor injuries that may not be otherwise noticed. People with diabetes are also more likely to sustain low-grade infections of the skin and to develop gangrene. Diabetics with foot problems occupy more hospital beds than diabetics with all other complications. In a survey of 70 diabetic patients carried out in the 1980s in the United Kingdom, 45 per cent were wearing shoes that were either too tight (37 per cent) or too loose (8 per cent). Improperly fitting shoes are thought to be an important factor in the aetiology of necrosis and ulceration in the diabetic foot, and the steam bath effect should be considered in both situations. Shampoo, if used frequently in the shower, can also cause considerable damage to the feet in diabetics.

Socks are meant to pad the foot inside the shoe and reduce any injury resulting from walking. Whereas in the past good woollen or cotton socks were always recommended, these tend to lose their size and shape after constant laundering. Recent work by sports' podiatrists in the United States has suggested that chunky, acrylic socks launder better, produce fewer blisters in athletes and are said to 'wick away' the sweat from the surface of the skin better than either cotton or wool. In this case technology appears to have provided a better solution than the natural form.

Fashion

The modern fashion industry is often responsible for damage to the skin by promoting clothing which does not protect against the elements, especially sunlight. It also promotes the wearing of high-heeled shoes in females, which constrict the feet and inflict trauma by being too tight and causing potentially damaging gait patterns. As a result, back and knee problems are not uncommon in women who regularly wear high-heeled shoes.

Is there such a thing as a 'bad hair day'?

What is jokingly referred to as a 'bad hair day' is probably founded in fact. Excessive sweat in the head results from the abundance of sweat glands in this part of the body and the fact that this may be the only part of the body protruding from an overly insulated bedding cover such as a doona. Sweat mixes with the natural 'grease' in the hair and forms a greasy mix (emulsion) which makes hair dull, lank and greasy.

Excessive shampooing and soaping thins the individual hairs (weathering) and results in a loss of 'bounce' and increased knotting. A 'bad hair day' therefore could be more than just a common cliché.

The fashion for having a tan encourages light skinned people to overexpose themselves to both natural and artificial forms of ultraviolet light. The consequences of this are seen in the form of excessive photo damage and skin cancer. Adequate sun protection should be the rule of the day. Sun filters and sun protective clothing are technology's answer to this, but these are only partially effective when social pressures entice users to believe that by using these products they can lie in the sun for longer. Damage still occurs in sunlight, proceeding to the development of tough, leathery, wrinkly skin in later life.

Chemicals

Modern household chemicals may have a useful role in helping us manage ourselves, our offices and our households, but many of these also have great potential for damaging the skin. The guiding rule should be to use all chemicals with great care in the lowest possible quantity and concentration. For example, it's likely that the average person uses about 100 times the necessary amount of washing-up detergent when washing dishes. Often this is complicated by wearing occlusive gloves made of modern synthetic materials which allow the hands to be inserted into much hotter water than usual. The resultant overheating and excessive sweating of the hands within the gloves can cause dermatitis of the hands which will not respond to the usual therapies. A more preferable option is to use the minimum amount of detergent in comfortably warm water, without gloves, but with the hands protected by a layer of moisturiser. Once the washing up is completed and the dishes stacked, the hands can be rinsed to remove any detergent present and some more moisturiser applied. If it is felt necessary, some boiling water can be poured over the dishes in order to 'sterilise' them without getting it on the hands. A similar attitude to other household chemicals is recommended.

7 Cleanliness and the skin

If the modern environment and modern technology are problems for the skin, what we do to counter these often just makes the skin problem worse. The immediate reaction for someone with dry skin, greasy hair and/or an itchy scalp is to have regular showers, scrub down with soap and shampoo the hair daily, repeatedly, often not realising that this is only drying the skin and scalp out more and leaving it open to that vicious cycle of dermatitis. There are a number of things we do that cause this to happen.

Showers and cleaning

Regular showering is good for the skin provided showers are brief and not too hot (pink skin in white-skinned people means the water is too hot). Strong soaps, however, tend to take away the surface layer of 'natural' grease on the skin, which is there to serve as a barrier function referred to previously. Washing with water only, on the other hand, dries out the epidermis and causes chapping, so we need some form of oil or grease as an alternative to soap. Simple and inexpensive moisturising lotion, the type that can be bought over the counter for a few dollars at any pharmacy, provides one solution to this, used both in the shower or bath and applied to the skin afterwards as an 'all-over' moisturiser.

It's important to recognise that it's not the bath or the shower

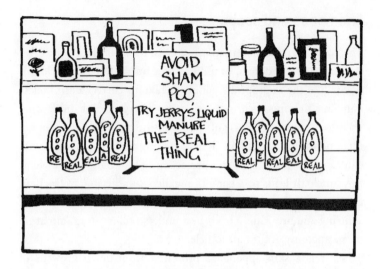

which is the problem for skin, but what's put in it—soaps and shampoos in particular. In the summer months in Australia this can become a real hazard because we often shower several times a day—after getting out of bed, after surfing or swimming, after exercise and often again before going to bed. Without the use of a moisturiser and/or an oil-based lotion for cleansing, the skin becomes more and more dry, opening itself up for environmental insult in the manner described in Chapter 3. If, on top of this drying, the skin is exposed to sunlight and salt water as is often the case in the summer months, the chances of insult through further drying are increased.

In the home environment as we've seen, rubber gloves are often used to protect the hands against dishwashing detergents. But while these provide some protection from the detergent, they can cause the hands to sweat and this tends to accumulate at the tips of the fingers, even with cotton gloves inside, resulting in fissuring and scaling of the finger pulps and damage to the nails.

Shampoos and soaps

The ads tell us that shampoos are a must for lovely hair. And after sleeping under a doona, or a night in a smoke filled nightclub, it seems like the appropriate action to take to correct dull, lifeless hair. But shampoo is a form of strong detergent, not unlike that used to 'scrape' the grease off plates in the dishwashing (can you imagine washing your hair in dishwashing detergent?). As such it can cause drying of the outer protective cells of the hair, known as the cuticle. It leads to a condition called 'weathering' of the hair, consisting of thinning of the individual hairs, increased tangling, splitting and breaking. This is best understood by an examination of the anatomy of the hair follicle.

Hair is a skin appendage produced from down growths of epidermis into the dermis (see Chapter 2). Not all animals have hair, but most mammals have some, even if only rudimentary. Humans have varied patterns of hair growth differing between males and females, and different families seem to inherit different mosaic patterns of hair growth.

Hair grows in cycles that vary from site to site. The average scalp hair grows for approximately four years and then falls out, to be replaced by another hair. The length of the hair cycle at other sites is usually related to the coarseness of the hair. Hair growth varies from decade to decade of life, and is controlled by hormonal activity, immunological and nutritional factors.

The individual hair grows from a hair matrix in the deep dermis which is surrounded by a complex of small blood vessels. It is usually associated with some pigment cells and consists of a cortex (shaft) surrounded by cuticle cells. During its passage up the hair follicle, the hair is surrounded by a number of protective layers called *root sheaths* which fall off as the hair approaches the

Differences between shampoo and conditioner

- Modern shampoos contain strong synthetic 'detergents'. A detergent is 'a substance which removes grease and dirt from a surface'. These are necessary for the removal of the thick, tacky emulsion formed by the mixture of a little scalp grease and excessive sweat.
- The detergent chemicals in shampoo produce 'bubbles' which are assumed by many consumers to be a sign of efficacy.
- It is virtually impossible to buy a gentle, non-detergent shampoo today—despite the description on the label.
- Conditioners contain substances known as 'surfactants' which are basically 'spreading agents'. There are several classes of these, some of which have mild detergent capacity sufficient for the cleansing of normal hair grease.
- Such surfactants are more gentle on the surface of the hair and skin than detergents, and can be used as often as desired without causing harm.

surface. The hair is virtually dead from the moment it leaves the cuticle cells.

As the hair grows above the level of the skin, it consists only of a *cortex* and *cuticle*, the latter being made up of many shield-like cells overlapping each other like scales on a fish, to protect the cortex (see diagram 7.1). The colour of the hair is dependent on pigment cells in the cortex and variation in pigmentation of the cortex gives rise to the well-known greying or whitening of hair which occurs with age and in other situations. Early greying, which can occur relatively

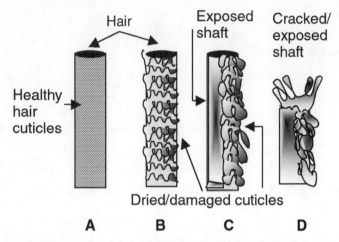

Hair

Exposed
shaft

Cracked/
exposed
shaft

Healthy
hair
cuticles

Dried/damaged cuticles

A   B   C   D

Diagram 7.1 The process of 'weathering' of the hair through over-shampooing

quickly, is often a familial trait and has some relationship in some people with the potential for diabetes. The 'sheen' of hair is dependent on a little grease and the uniform reflection of light from a healthy cuticle. It might sound fanciful, but it's not unrealistic to suggest that skin problems on the feet, such as tinia, could have their origin in the overuse of shampoo for the hair!

Washing hair with detergent-like shampoos tends to disrupt the cuticle cells on the outside of the hairs. They no longer fit tightly over one another, and this enables the shampoo to penetrate between the cuticles cells and attack the body of the cortex. It also causes the cuticle cells to reflect light differently, and give the hair a dull look. The hair can knot and tangle more easily as a result, and this can lead to increased breakage of hairs, and is often referred to as 'split ends'. This whole process, which is typically referred to as 'weathering' of the hair, is shown in the progression from a healthy to a damaged hair shaft from diagram A to D in diagram 7.1.

The famous French dermatologist Dr Aron-Brunetiere has likened shampoo to industrial strength detergent. It 'scrapes' the natural grease out of hair and can cause damage to the hair, scalp, face, shoulders and upper trunk, hands—and even the feet if hair is regularly shampooed under the shower.

It's difficult to tell from an ingredients list just how strong a shampoo may be. In any case, even so-called 'gentle' versions can damage the epidermal barrier of the scalp sufficiently to make the skin more vulnerable to irritation, while having little positive long-term benefit for the hair. The biggest problem for most women is that after shampooing and drying their hair, either with a towel or hair dryer, it looks light and attractive again. But this appearance only lasts for a few hours, after which it goes flat. The only way to make it look 'bouncy' again is to repeat the process. And each time this is done, the individual hairs are damaged further.

Some experts suggest that while grease can be removed quite easily from the hair by combing, brushing or even towelling, when it is mixed with an excessive amount of sweat, such as after a night of sleeping under a doona as described previously, emulsification takes place. This causes a thick, greasy, tacky substance to be deposited on the hair that is difficult to remove without the use of more and more detergent shampoos. It finally causes 'stringy' hair which is incapable of being repaired. And the process of dealing with it becomes a cyclical one.

Hair can be easily managed by using conditioner alone. Conditioners contain surfactants (spreading agents), some of which have mild detergent capacities, enough to remove the normal grease in the hair but not enough to remove the thick tacky emulsion mentioned above. The only way to prevent the formation of this emulsion is to stop overheating at night. Conditioners can be used as often as desired because the level of detergent activity is much less than in shampoo. It is important to use a lot of conditioner (about two tablespoons), however, and to rinse the hair well. During the transition period from shampoo to conditioner some increase in greasiness may be noted, perhaps along with a little itching and flaking, but this usually settles in a matter of weeks. The condition of the hair becomes noticeably better by the end of six to eight weeks— provided overheating at night is avoided.

Soap is also an overused commodity in the modern world. Soap is made from oil and alkalines. It works by washing the grease, or sebum, off the skin and in the process changing it from its usual slightly acid state to one of alkalinity. Unfortunately no soap made has been able to differentiate between the skin's natural oils and exogenous dirt. Thus, washing with soap always involves the removal of the uppermost layer of oil from the skin, as well as changing the skin from predominantly acid to alkaline. Yeasts, fungi and some forms of bacteria, especially gastro-intestinal bacteria, grow better in alkaline situations and hence this is a recipe for bacterial 'insult' to the skin.

Most dermatologists now agree that we wash for comfort, not for health. In the words of one such expert:

> ... all soaps are potentially damaging to the skin. Modern middle class people are too obsessed with cleanliness. Less washing is better. The skin doesn't care whether it is clean or not—unlike in former days when dirty skin spread contagion.
>
> Wolf R. Clinics in Dermatology, 1996

'Moisturising' soaps

Traditionally these soaps, which often contain glycerine as humectant (water-holding compound), were popular in places such as Lebanon, where every family seemed to have its own recipe, and in Marseilles which gave its name to such soaps. Their use is of intermediate value only since they tend to perpetuate the idea of scrubbing the skin. They are less effective than the use of moisturising cream and water as set out in the final chapter of this book. Grease can be satisfactorily removed from the skin by dissolving it in another grease which dissolves in water.

Saline baths

Baths containing salt, Condy's crystals, baking soda and a range of other such 'elixirs' have been traditionally used in the past for the treatment of certain skin diseases, particularly if these were 'weeping'. However, in the main these also tend to dry out the skin and have no long-term benefits.

Oatmeal baths

As a skin cleansing agent, skin sedative and soap substitute, oatmeal has been used for thousands of years. It is said to have been popular among the ancient Egyptians. There have been many modifications of the original technique in order to make it more attractive, to prevent plumbing problems (in clogging up the drain), and to modify it for use as a soap bar, but none seems to be as effective as the original routine of bathing in oatmeal itself. When oatmeal enclosed in a stocking or muslin bag is added to water, a soft white mucousy substance (mucin) is exuded which will cleanse the skin adequately without damaging it, oil it slightly and make it feel much less 'angry'. Hence the use of oatmeal is one practice which is generally looked on favourably by dermatologists.

The details for oatmeal baths are found in the summary in Chapter 10 of this book.

Scrubbing and drying

It is better to treat skin with tender loving care rather than to scrub it, and to waterproof it rather than to dry it out. Physical damage should always be kept to a minimum. The fetish of making sure that all skin is dry is a relic from the past. If skin is adequately waterproofed it can look after itself. Drying talcum powder, for example, tends to collect in skin creases and become abrasive. Scrubbing the skin with a towel and the aggressive use of scourers such as loofahs belongs in the field of masochism and has no real role in skin care.

The proponents of such practices maintain that the skin needs assistance in exfoliation in order to remain healthy.

Hair dryers

Although hair dryers in themselves are not as damaging as may be thought, their excessive use can contribute to hair damage. If the hair is in good order, the cuticle protects the cortex against waterlogging. If the cuticle is badly damaged, the hair cortex takes up more water and takes longer to dry out. One useful way of reducing the use of the hair dryer is to firstly dry the hair with a synthetic chamois. These can be obtained expensively as sports towels, or more cheaply from the car maintenance section of your local supermarket. It will remove the bulk of the moisture quickly, particularly if the hair is long and thick. If a dryer is still necessary after this, it can be used relatively briefly at a mild temperature so it is less likely to damage the hair follicle.

Deodorants, antiperspirants and aftershave

Deodorants and aftershave lotions are further products of marketing gimmickry. Where a new approach to caring for the skin such as discussed in these pages is undertaken, there is usually no longer the need to use deodorant. The people who *need* deodorant are those who use soap. The people who *sell* deodorant are usually those who sell soap. It is possible that the regular use of soap brings about minor alterations in the composition of the bacterial flora which are normally resident on the skin, in turn giving rise to changes in body odour. And while this might call for a deodorant to counteract the effect, it would seem wiser to not produce the effect in the first place. Most excessive body odour results from wearing unwashed clothing for a number of days. Discreet enquiries of patients has revealed that though outer garments may be changed daily, underclothes are not necessarily changed so frequently!

Antiperspirants work by blocking the outer portion of the sweat duct. This forms a physical barrier from which sweat is unable to escape to the outer surface of the skin, where it would normally be evaporated and hence aid in heat loss. Perspiration (sweat) is of course most common as a response to environmental temperatures and the heat produced by the body during physical exertion. It serves the natural function of cooling the body, without which we would continue to overheat until we 'burst a boiler'. Although there are some idiosyncratic smells associated with individual sweat, the main offensive smells that come from it result from all those approaches to soaping, drying and cleansing that we have discussed so far, and which make the body respond in an 'unnatural' way. It seems ironic that antiperspirant marketers typically use top level athletes—who make a sizeable living these days out of good, healthy sweat—to try to encourage the rest of us not to put up with something which would not be offensive if we didn't do the things the marketers continually try to convince us to do. Perceived discomfort from excessive sweating is often associated with stress and occurs mainly in shaved armpits. It can be reduced by aluminium salts in deodorants. However, allergy to such salts is common.

'Aftershave' lotions usually have alcoholic or astringent bases which make the skin feel 'taught and terrific' on application. If perfumes are added to these there's a common belief that they'll also have some sexual attraction (at least if the ads are to be believed). The bases in aftershave can damage the skin over a long period, making it tough and leather-like. Some of the perfumes can also induce sensitivity to sunlight and produce pigmentation. It is far better to apply a little moisturiser to the facial skin after shaving than to try to suffer in macho style from the stinging effect of an aftershave lotion.

Cosmetics

In general, cosmetics have little overall effect on the skin. But the damage inflicted on the skin by some cosmetics or medicaments can be a problem for some women. Various combinations of showering, shampooing, cleansing and drying mentioned above are capable of aggravating, augmenting and prolonging any instability already present in the skin. Adding a cosmetic which may consist of dozens of ingredients, thus raising the chances of one or a combination of ingredients to which the skin may be sensitive, can result in skin insult and dermatitis in some form. Quite often this leads to medicines being prescribed for the skin but, unless the causes are considered in their own right, medicines are unlikely to have any long-term effect. Indeed, they may just add to the problem because of the addition of yet another potential skin irritant.

Much facial dermatitis, periorbital irritation and inflammation, and much of the so-called adult acne of today which fails to respond to standard acne treatments is the result of external damage inflicted on the skin. These problems are often aggravated by the drying effects of agents such as toners, tonics, exfoliants and other cosmetics. And while few would support the total elimination of cosmetics in women, there is a definite case to be made for careful and perceptive use. Skin problems which may appear to be totally unrelated by virtue of timing or localisation may indeed have a causal basis in some cosmetic products. Fragrances in cosmetics are the most frequent cause of cosmetic allergy, both from products primarily used for their scent (perfumes, colognes, eaux de toilette, aftershave and deodorants) and from other scented products.

Most allergic reactions to cosmetics are caused by cosmetics that remain on the skin, such as skin care products, hair cosmetics (most notably hair dyes), nail cosmetics (polish, hardener), deodorants and other perfumes and facial and eye make-up. 'Rinse off' or 'wash off' products such as soap, shampoo, bath foam and shower foam rarely cause contact allergic reactions.

'Natural' cosmetics

In general, the more chemicals put on the skin at the same time, the greater the chances of skin damage occurring as a result of irritation and allergy. Most so-called 'natural' products are mixtures of many ingredients which vary from time to time depending on the season of the year and the time of harvest of the product. Lanolin, from sheep's wool, is often claimed to have particular benefits for the skin because it is a 'natural' product. Yet lanolins are known to contain over 60 different components and thus have a relatively high potential for skin reactions. Most plant extracts also consist of many ingredients and the fact that these are 'natural' is little different to a product consisting of exactly the same chemicals made up in a laboratory. There's also the question of consistency. Unless each batch of 'natural' products is rigorously analysed before being used, it is almost impossible to have uniformity in these products. They therefore have a greater potential for causing harm than products with more limited, preferably inert ingredients

The advantage of using synthesised chemicals (which have most often been discovered in plants anyway) is that the exact

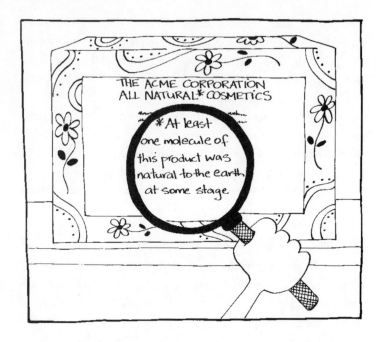

formulation is known and can be better controlled. It may be possible to get away with using so-called 'natural' cosmetics, but the potential for adverse reactions is always present and possibly to a greater extent in natural products than those made by experienced chemists. An even better preference would be to use a mixture of water and paraffins (para = little; affinity = attraction), which have little attraction to other substances and are thus virtually inert, made up into a simple lotion or cream with the minimal amount of preservatives to prevent bacterial contamination.

Other 'natural' products

The term 'natural' has unfortunately been abused by marketers in recent times. This is unfortunate because down through the ages, and still today, 'natural' products can be used to great effect in many forms of medicine, including dermatology. Local aloe veras, for example, are currently being used to good effect by dermatologists in Africa as inexpensive treatments for skin infection, psoriasis, genital herpes, and as a sunscreen for those with sensitive skin. But the fact that this may have some value in at least some of these conditions doesn't guarantee that aloe vera can cure everything from ingrown toenails to plantar warts, as is often claimed by over-zealous promoters of natural products.

On the other side of the fence, experienced and skilful chemists are able to synthesise substances produced in the body such as elastins and collagens which hold skin cells together and give them their elasticity. But being able to reproduce these, and introduce them into the body, doesn't guarantee a response similar to that which occurs when these substances are produced physiologically. Synthetic products can have just as many unknown effects as the 'natural' ones.

There are obviously lessons to be learned from both the 'natural' and 'synthetic' product advocates. The modern pharmaceutical industry has attempted to find the most important and effective constituents of many natural products, examine their structure and synthesise them in a pure form, before presenting them for sale in pharmaceutical products. This may work, but it also may ignore the potentially powerful effects of ingredient combinations in the natural product. Natural health specialists can adopt a product for use on the basis of its effect in traditional societies but, equally, this can overlook the powerful effect of tradition and ritual in medicinal treatments. 'Pointing the bone' can have a fatal effect on a tribal Aboriginal, but it might only serve to make a non-Indigenous person hungry, or fall about laughing.

Finally, it's worth commenting about the supposed purity of 'natural' products. Some of the most potent poisons known are 'natural'—plant and animal. Also, while the natural ingredients of a lot of plants can be beneficial for many people, they too can be harmful for others. Camomile tea, for example, while generally a healthy alternative to normal caffeinated teas for most people, can contain a 'belladonna-like' substance which can cause hallucinations in a small number of sensitive people. An interesting tale from artistic history also illustrates this point: the artist Vincent Van Gogh was famous for his paintings with yellow halos around them for which, at the time, there seemed little explanation. It was only realised later that Van Gogh used the plant foxglove, which contains digitalis (still used today as a heart medication) and was used as a treatment for the epilepsy from which he suffered. We now know that one of the other chemicals in foxglove can modify the retina of the eye and lead a person to see objects with yellow halos around them. Hence, while foxglove has known advantages in certain instances, it also has hitherto unrecognised side effects. This emphasises the need to keep an open (and cynical) mind, about both 'natural' and manufactured products.

8 Medications—good effects and side effects

The human body is a complex organism. And while we've probably learned more about the way it functions over the last two to three decades than in the whole of human history, we are still a long way from a definitive understanding. One thing we do know is that all external medications, be they 'natural' or 'synthetic', used to correct health problems in the body can have side effects. In some cases these are minor (some are never even noticed), and are part of the *cost* that has to be borne by someone who is profiting from the *benefits* of medication. Others can be quite severe, in some cases more unsettling than the problem itself. In this case we would have to wonder about the value of using any such medication. The art of using medication is to achieve a positive balance (more benefit than cost) as the 'bottom line', so it is important for anyone using medication to understand both the supposed advantages and potential side effects of that medication.

There are many different patterns of reaction to drugs that can come out in the skin. Dermatologists spend a good deal of their time trying to sort out such reactions, and while some of these might be truly allergic responses to one or more ingredients in the medication, others can have a less clear cut causality. If there is a reaction, a whole range of factors need to be considered, including:

- the disease for which the drug is being used;
- other drugs being used (interactions);
- whether the drug has been used previously and for how long;
- whether an underlying condition is involved;
- how troublesome the reaction is;
- how important the drug is; and
- if any substitute drug could be used with less chance of a similar reaction.

There are obvious dangers in unnecessarily stopping a helpful drug and replacing it with a less effective drug, or one with greater potential for side effects. There are also problems in assuming an adverse reaction from a medication based on a previous history. For example, twenty or thirty years ago some people were told that they were allergic to penicillin. Yet re-challenging these people with a newer form of penicillin under strict supervision can sometimes show that this is not necessarily true for all penicillins today. If the earlier findings are taken as immutable, this could result in the elimination of a valuable form of therapy in cases where it may prove vital for a quick and effective benefit.

It's also not uncommon for someone on medication to take fright at the appearance of a harmless rash after a day or so, and stop the medication immediately as a result. But this may be one of the relatively minor costs that needs to be paid to achieve the benefits of a good medication. The skill is in deciding just by how much the benefits exceed the costs, if at all, and hence whether the medication is worth the trouble. Some general medications with more entries on the cost side of the skin ledger are listed below. This is followed by a list of potentially beneficial skin treatments.

Treatments with potentially harmful side effects

Although the medications mentioned here can have some negative side effects on the skin, it is advisable to always consult a doctor before discontinuing medication. Immediately ceasing the use of these drugs may, in some cases, be life threatening.

Cortisone creams

Among the more common skin applications are the cortisone creams. These can be very effective in reducing inflammation, stopping itching and making the skin more comfortable; that is, suppressing *symptoms*. On the other hand, they *cure* nothing. Nor are they meant to. Their dermatological function is to suppress reactions so that proper healing can take place. Using cortisone is like using an umbrella in the rain: it won't stop the rain, but it might make you more comfortable getting from A to B while it's raining. These creams can buy time while a skin condition burns itself out, or the real causes are eliminated.

On the downside, the intermittent use of cortisones can make skin diseases worse through a 'rebound' effect, which can occur if there is no attempt to eradicate the real cause of the problem. The overuse of cortisone can cause skin thinning, the increased dilatation of blood vessels (due to the rebound effect), the development of stretch marks and easy bruising and the perpetuation of skin infections. Like all medications, the costs and benefits of cortisone creams need to be carefully considered before they are used to treat problems of the skin. Some areas of the skin are more vulnerable to adverse reactions than others to strong cortisone creams. The face, the groin, the insides of the thighs and beneath the breasts are the main areas where this occurs. Red faces and stretch marks on the insides of the thighs and breasts are examples of this.

Lanolin

As we have noted before, the quickest way to make the skin allergic to something is to apply a multiplicity of different chemicals to it at the one time. Intermittent applications over a long period can also have the same effect. In the past, lanolin and many other so-called 'natural' substances have been used on the skin. But lanolin, which comes from sheep's wool, contains over 60 different components (it has been described as 'a wolf in sheep's clothing'), and hence the chances of an allergic reaction to any one or combination of these components are higher than they would be to other medications. There are no major advantages of lanolin over a simpler moisturising cream purchased inexpensively over the counter at a pharmacy.

Cholesterol-lowering agents

Cholesterol is a waxy, fatty like substance (not a true 'fat') which is carried in the blood and is an important constituent of cell membranes, especially in the epidermis. As such, cholesterol is a vital component of human physiology. But too much of it, and particularly too much of the more dense versions of its molecule, can lead to the deterioration of blood vessels and possible heart disease. For this reason cholesterol-lowering medication is widely prescribed, often with little consideration of any potential side effects.

There's little doubt that cholesterol-lowering drugs can be lifesavers under appropriate circumstances. But because cholesterol is important in the functioning of skin cells, high doses of cholesterol-lowering medication can sometimes lead to itchy skin disorders if continued for long periods. Some people, with appropriate encouragement and a change in diet, are able to stop the medication once cholesterol is reduced to a 'normal' level. Still, pharmaceutical manufacturers gain little by this practice and so there is often little education or incentive to either reduce the medication totally, or at least reduce its strength. Regular blood checks should be made, together with changes in diet and lifestyle designed to reduce cholesterol. By doing this, it may be possible to avoid some of the dermatological downsides of an otherwise effective cardiovascular medication. Hair loss—thinning and fracture of the individual hairs—is not uncommon with these drugs.

Antibiotics and antiseptics

When antibiotics are taken to deal with infection they have effects on every part of the body, including the skin. The skin has a normal resident population of bacteria, most of which are benign but most important to the proper health and functioning of the skin. These help to control transient aggressive bacteria which are usually on the skin in small numbers. When either antibiotics or antiseptics are used in excess, the benign bugs tend to be more vulnerable and so are more easily eliminated, leaving the playing field open to be occupied by the more aggressive bacteria, especially those that have developed resistance to antibiotics and antiseptics.

Broad spectrum antibiotics can upset the delicate balance between bacteria and Candida (thrush) normally present in the bowel. If an overload of Candida in the bowel occurs, it may give rise to mild increases in flatulence and increased intestinal movement, even to the extent of producing diarrhoea. The lower parts of the body, particularly around the anus and vagina, become swamped with Candida, which may establish itself in areas with a low resistance, giving rise to persistent itch. The application of anti-Candidal medications to these areas may kill off the local Candida, but do nothing about the continuing supply of organisms from the bowel. Oral Nystatin is not very popular on the basis that it is not absorbed from the bowel and so cannot help in such a situation. Nevertheless, it is a very safe drug which does reduce the intestinal overload (including the symptoms), and by reducing the recurring contamination of the peri-anal and vaginal areas goes a long way to preventing the well-known recurrences.

The current tendency to overuse antibiotics produces a great number of different skin problems, but probably most important is the result of not allowing the skin to look after itself. The outcome of this can be seen in the photo section. Facial redness in 5a resulted from a combination of overheating and overuse of antibiotics to deal with this. Picture 5b shows the effects of de-heating and eliminating antibiotics.

The ability of the skin to cope with infections is something which has to be learned by the skin over a period of time. If this learning is suppressed, that learning never takes place. Care should therefore be taken in the use of both antibiotics and antiseptics (some of which are quite corrosive on the skin) in order to ensure that the 'bottom line' in this case remains 'in the black'.

Heart medications

All heart medications have some side effects, far too numerous to list in detail. For this reason, many people with blood pressure problems and other heart conditions probably have to try three or four different medications before finding the most suitable one for them.

Check with the prescribing doctor if skin problems are noticed while on any particular heart medication.

Antidepressants and other psychotropic medications

For reasons explained previously, some of the earlier drugs used as antidepressants started life as antihistamines (used in the treatment of skin disease to reduce itch, hives etc.). These are often known as anti-allergy drugs. They therefore can have a useful place in the management of skin disorders, but when used in high doses can give rise to variations in sweating, produce a very dry mouth and cause other side effects.

Many psychotropic drugs have a potential to initiate photo-sensitivity (an increased sensitivity to sunlight). Other medications in common use, such as lithium carbonate, can aggravate or initiate skin problems (such as psoriasis). In such cases compromise has to be used if the person is to continue benefiting from the use of this drug.

One again, we need to reinforce the statement that all drugs are like pennies with two sides, having advantages and disadvantages. The skin is often a window for such disadvantages, giving rise to the production of large catalogues on drug-induced eruptions, their types, frequency and interactions. All drugs, including vitamins, minerals and herbal remedies (most of these have a multiplicity of known and unknown constituents, each with its own potential for producing adverse reactions), can be beneficial, but they can also cause harm and this is often manifest first in the skin. Our constant aim should be to gain the benefits from medication while keeping the costs to a minimum. Keep the bottom line black—compromise.

AHA (alpha hydroxy acids)

AHAs have become very popular recently as a result of reports suggesting that these rejuvenate the skin. The proposed mechanism for this is through repeated peeling. AHAs are derived from fruit acids, and have been used over the centuries in their cruder form (such as lemon juice) for this purpose. If skin is continually peeled, its ability to deal with sunlight is reduced and hence the prospects of skin damage from the sun are increased. Recently, cosmetics companies have begun to add AHAs to many of their products in what seems an indiscriminate fashion. This has prompted the American Food and Drug Administration (FDA) to question the propriety of this practice in the United States, but their findings have not yet been reported. In the meantime, there seems to be no great long-term benefit to the individual from such products and there may be some harm caused by them.

Self treatments that can help the skin

Throughout much of this book we have been critical of the manufacture and over-promotion of many skin treatments. This is largely because of the inaccurate and often unsupported way in which these have been advertised to the public. It is not meant to imply that all skin care products should be cast in the same league. There are some very helpful products on the market, and although none can fulfil the promise of a new skin as is suggested in advertising by the super-models, they can assist the changes in lifestyle recommended here by allowing the skin an effective environment in which to recover. Examples of these are listed below.

Moisturisers

Skin moisturisers work not, as the name implies, by adding moisture to the skin, but by preventing this from being lost through heat and dryness. This is like the polish on a dining room table which is designed to maintain the inherent condition of the wood by providing a protective layer on the surface. If the surface dries out, moisture is likely to be lost from the deeper layers of timber and this will cause fissuring and cracking of the wood and a decline in overall condition. It makes little sense to incessantly scrub and rub the surface with abrasive chemicals, just as it makes little sense to scour the body and hair with soaps and detergents, particularly if the surface is not then 'polished' to prevent further damage.

Moisturisers in skin care products come in many forms. However, the main distinguishing characteristic between most is the price. A basic moisturiser requires little more than a simple protective, non-oily base which can be purchased in the generic form as sorbolene cream (with added glycerol) from any chemist. Because this is generic, the price for a large jar (500g) is usually less than $5. In contrast, commercially promoted moisturisers, which can range from $60 to $200 for a small quantity, have an image of effectiveness based on price—the more expensive it is, the more effective it is thought to be. In reality, the extra expense is really only for advertising, packaging and in some cases added constituents of dubious benefit with some perfume. The more constituents, the greater the chance of an adverse reaction. In a 'blind' trial carried out recently by the Australian Consumer's Association, sorbolene cream was rated as good as, or more effective than, more expensive cosmetics moisturisers when these were packaged in indistinguishable containers.

The extra money paid for moisturising creams with vitamins (not absorbed by the skin anyway) or made from 'natural' substances is unnecessary, as it is the base in these products, rather than the additions, that provides the moisturising qualities.

Sunscreens

Sunscreens have special chemical ingredients which prevent the harmful ultraviolet light (UVL) rays of the sun from reaching the skin. Because it is the UVL rays which cause the initial redness and later reaction of the skin to sunlight, these creams are thought to have a potential value (although not to the extent of allowing unlimited sun exposure without danger). Sun damage is also

How do sunscreens work?

Sunscreens were originally developed in the 1920s. There are two main types: one forms a physical barrier which resists penetration by the sun's harmful ultraviolet rays (e.g. zinc creams and those containing titanium dioxide). The second, and more common, type presents a chemical barrier which changes the harmful rays and deflects them back into the environment. This is rated using a system called SPF (skin protection factor) which is a loose measurement of the time taken on average skin to cause an erythema (reddening of the skin). An SPF of 15 suggests a minimum time of 15 minutes. However, this does not indicate an SPF of 30 is twice as 'strong'. An SPF of 15 may allow only 7 per cent of the harmful rays through, whereas an SPF of 30 would allow less e.g. 3 per cent.

thought to be the prime factor in accelerated skin aging, possibly through the development of free radicals in skin tissue, which hasten the aging process, and so sunscreens might also have the potential for slowing signs of aging.

The effectiveness of a screen is based on an index called its SPF, or sun protection factor, which is a loosely based estimate of the multiple of the time taken for reddening of the skin compared to exposure in a standard light source without a sunscreen. An SPF of 5, for example, means when worn it would take five times the normal length of time before burning. An SPF of 15 simply means it takes three times as long for the screen to become ineffective as with an SPF of 5. Screens with a maximum SPF of 30 are now available and are recommended for anyone who spends long periods of time exposed to the sun.

Some recent findings show that sunscreens may do more than just shield the skin. Some Australian research showed that among fair-skinned people not only did those who used a sunscreen with an SPF of 17 develop fewer skin cancers than those who used a placebo lotion, but their existing skin cancers were more likely to go into remission. As a caution, sunscreens should not be used as licence for uncontrolled exposure. They can have allergic effects in sensitive people and should also be carefully applied if used during outdoor endurance events such as fun-runs.

An important rider to the use of sunscreens is the recent finding that some of these may cause photo contact allergy in some susceptible people. Sometimes this can be overlooked because the symptoms may be interpreted as the failure of the sunscreen to adequately protect against the sun's rays rather than as an adverse reaction. If regular reactions occur to sunscreens, these should be tested for allergic properties before continuing to be used.

And as mentioned earlier, it is also very helpful to MOVE while in the sun!

Emulsifying ointment

Paraffin tends to be simple and almost inert. Preparations such as emulsifying ointment BP can be very effective as a general daily moisturiser. They need to be mixed with water until creamy and then applied thinly to the skin. Frequent small applications are better than occasional excesses.

Tea tree oil

Tea tree oil has been used in Australia as an antiseptic by Indigenous people for thousands of years. Only recently, however, has this been proven to have some antiseptic properties. Research carried out at the University of Western Australia has proven the presence of several antibacterial substances in the oil which could help explain its effectiveness under certain circumstances. This may have value in the treatment and prevention of some skin lesions. However, tea tree oil can also be drying and irritating. It should therefore never be used as a form of 'blunderbuss' therapy on the skin.

Lip cream

Unlike many cosmetics, lip balm generally has a moisturising rather than a drying effect on the sensitive tissue of the lips. For this reason it can be helpful in stopping the lips from drying out. Lip balm also reduces the amount of 'lip licking' that often occurs sub-consciously and which can contribute to skin damage on the lips. Special sunscreen lip creams are especially useful as the sensitive skin on the lips and the way in which particularly the bottom lip is exposed to the sunlight make the lips particularly vulnerable to sun damage.

Foundation creams

These are generally used as a base for other cosmetics. And while the cosmetics themselves may have no real benefits (apart from aesthetically), and indeed may have potential costs for the skin, foundation creams can act as proxy moisturisers, sealing moisture in the skin. They may also have some benefit as sunscreens, reducing damage from sun exposure.

Retinoids

Retinoid creams, which are basically derivatives of vitamin A, became extremely popular as anti-aging agents in the early 1990s. Since that time their popularity has waned somewhat. One possible reason for this is that such treatments work largely through their inflammatory effect, and as such need to be continually applied.

They have not been convincingly shown to have a long-term 'curative' effect on the skin's aging. Retinoids are known to contain anti-oxidants, however, which act against free radical molecules in the body and are known to be linked to aging. Retinoids can be very useful in the treatment of complicated skin disorders but their main use is well beyond the scope of this book.

9 Myths and fallacies about the skin

Like other areas of health, the field of dermatology is rife with mythology. Some of this has been around for eons and has been passed down through the ages without solid scientific or even practical evidence to support it. Other misinformation comes from commercial manufacturers who have their own products to push. Some of the more common myths around are illustrated in the examples outlined below.

There are seven layers of skin

It's not quite clear what this means. There are, in fact, three compartments which make up the skin: the epidermis, the dermis and the subcutaneous fat (see Chapter 2). The epidermis is the outer layer of the skin, which is constantly being renewed by migration of cells from the dermo-epidermal junction. It varies in thickness from area to area. The process of removing the 'dead' cells from the outer layer proceeds normally on its own in most people. Scrubbing off (exfoliating) the skin surface, which in the past has been popular and is now being revived, may have a place in certain circumstances but its widespread, uncritical use is not to be recommended. There is no practical value in the notion that the skin has seven layers.

The more hair is shampooed the nicer it looks

Over-shampooing can dry out the cuticle cells of the hair, which in healthy hair should be tightly packed and overlap each another like scales on a fish (see Chapter 8). Spaces open up between the cells with excessive shampooing, allowing the shampoo to penetrate into the body of the hair causing further damage through the process known as 'weathering'. With weathering, individual hairs become thinner and tangle more easily. They also break off and develop into what are commonly known as 'split ends'. This process can be temporarily disguised by the use of a lot of conditioner, and the hair may look healthy immediately after blow drying, but it begins to go flat and lose its bounce within a few hours. The only immediate way to restore the appearance is to re-shampoo and blow dry the hair. But this causes more damage and hair subjected to this form of repeated damage cannot be repaired. Its appearance can be disguised by coating it with mousse or other hair products, but this does not repair the situation. The only 'cure' is to perhaps shorten the hair, stop causing further damage and wait for the damaged hair to grow out at the painfully slow rate of about 1 centimetre per month. On this basis it usually takes five to six months to restore the bounce in the hair.

Hot showers help to cool you down

It's commonly thought that hot water, even on a hot day, will 'open' the pores of the skin and cool off the body. In reality, a hot shower causes perspiration which, if accompanied by excessive soaping and scouring, can actually be harmful. It is unlikely that skin 'pores' open and close as is generally imagined; I can't ever remember being 'winked at' by a pore! Hence a tepid shower is probably better than either a hot or cold shower. A hot shower followed by a cold shower, which is thought to be beneficial, has no value for the skin.

Saunas and steam baths are good for the skin

The most common belief about heat treatments such as saunas and steam baths is that they help reduce weight. However, it's now well known that any weight loss by these methods is from fluid, through sweat, which is replaced immediately on rehydration. Recent research does show that saunas may have some value in recovery from vigorous exercise in top-level athletes. They can also provide a psychological feeling of wellbeing, which shouldn't be undervalued. However, they have little or no value in 'cleansing' the skin. Indeed, in young children (who have an increased skin area compared with adults and are more vulnerable to the effects of overheating) and in the elderly they can be potentially dangerous. This is especially so where cardiac problems exist. Heat treatments tend to lower the blood pressure, then a cold shower (or roll in the snow in the case of the Scandinavians) can raise it dramatically as the arteries contract suddenly to preserve heat. Where there are inherent heart problems this presents a dangerous combination. Even in Finland, where there is said to be one sauna for every four members of the population, the benefit of the practice is now being questioned.

Anyone with olive skin has oily skin

There is a common misconception that olive and oily skin go together. Most people from the Mediterranean, the Middle East and the northern parts of Asia have olive skin, but their skin is actually very dry. Very few people, if any, have 'oily' skin. As a result olive-skinned people can also get skin cancer, even though they may have a little less tendency than fair-skinned Caucasians to do so. Also, contrary to popular belief, the consumption of olive oil on a regular basis, while possibly having some benefits in the prevention of heart disease, is unlikely to increase skin oiliness.

Dark-skinned people can't get skin cancer

There's little doubt that the incidence of skin cancer in darker races is less than that in Caucasians. However, dark-skinned people are not entirely immune, as is often thought. Melanoma in coloured people is mainly found on the less pigmented areas of the body such as the palms of the hands and soles of the feet and underneath the nails, and it is often of a very aggressive type.

You catch a cold by being in the cold or getting wet

Viral infections occur when immunity is low. The virus enters the body, and then spends a few days (the incubation period) multiplying before it is released into the circulation in the process called *viraemia*. Viraemia is accompanied by a sudden peak in temperature followed by a rapid fall, which is associated with a feeling of 'chill' and possibly shivering and rigors. After this, the viral infection proceeds in a normal manner and slowly resolves with some improvement in the body's immunity. It is probably because of this feeling of chill that we speak of 'colds' and 'chills' and for this reason cold or wet is often thought of as the cause of such a 'cold'.

It must be remembered that infection was present for some days before the viraemia occurred and the cause of such infection may therefore be unrelated to the cold. Colds and flu are more common in the colder winter months because of the greater opportunity for spread when people are confined more closely indoors to avoid the cold.

Most hives are due to allergy

It has often been assumed that hives result from an allergy to food, insect bites or other external factors. It's now realised that there can be many other physical, emotional or chemical causes, and that perhaps no more than 25 per cent of hives are actually caused by allergy. Histamine, which is released as a response to the introduction of an unrecognised intruder in the body, causes the dilatation of small blood vessels in the dermis, which allows fluid to escape into the tissue causing 'weals'. This also gives rise to the sensation of itch. Some medications such as aspirin can cause hives by both allergic and chemical release of histamine. Skin which is dry and sensitive can react even to stroking with a fingernail with man-made (factitious) weals and in this case scratch and prick tests for allergy need to be interpreted with caution. Heat, cold, water, the release of acetyl choline prior to sweating and many other factors singly or in combination can also cause hives, in the absence of an allergic reaction.

All the bugs have to be soaped off the skin

The skin has a normal population of bacteria well accustomed to living there and together doing a good job in keeping the skin healthy. The competition between the 'good' and 'bad' bugs achieves a state of equilibrium which is healthy for skin. And while we all have a small population of 'bad' bugs, the competition usually maintains this at a very low level. The use of soaps, antiseptics and medicated chemicals on the skin tends to alter the balance of the bugs and often kills many of the 'goodies', allowing the 'baddies' to take over. In many cases, people who substitute sorbolene cream for soap find they no longer have a need to use deodorant.

Antiseptic is good in the bath

In 'caring' for children, many parents will follow the instructions on the label of some antiseptics and add a few drops to the bath each day. Unfortunately, this has little positive value and can actually lead to allergic reactions to some of the constituents in the antiseptic. There is no value in dicing with the mix of ingredients contained in such products, particularly when there is no obvious advantage in doing so.

A 'nice' body smell is the smell of a good deodorant

Over the years we have been indoctrinated to ply the skin with soaps and other chemicals, and in doing so increasing body odour by changing the bacterial balance on the skin. The general response to this has been to try to counter it by the use of deodorants, so we have become accustomed to thinking that unless one smells of a deodorant one has an unacceptable body odour. Perhaps the worst situation is a mixture of odour from clothing which is being worn for a second or third day or week in combination with a highly perfumed deodorant—the full catastrophe! Changing clothing regularly and keeping the body well moisturised is enough to remove more offensive smells. The discomfort of sweat dripping out of a shaved armpit is exaggerated by the hair having been removed. This can be alleviated by an antiperspirant, but this can have allergic effects.

If an aftershave or an antiseptic stings, it's good for the skin

Market research in the United States has shown that unless an aftershave or antiseptic 'stings' it's thought by consumers to have no value. This is based on the 'no pain, no gain' philosophy which has no basis in fact. The use of these substances can cause dermatitis and changes in pigmentation due to the action of the sun on some of their constituents. Hence it's not necessary, and indeed may be unwise, to go for a product that provides a 'bite'.

A tan equates with being healthy

A suntan can promote a psychological feeling of wellbeing in some people, but contrary to popular belief it has no positive benefit for health. Melanin, the skin pigment that causes skin to go dark after exposure to sunlight, is not as effective as was once thought in the prevention of further skin damage, particularly when tested against the effects of modern sunscreens.

Skin should be kept dry i.e. with baby powder

The bulk of this book has been based around dismissing the idea that dryness is good for skin. The idea of keeping the skin dry, especially in babies, has been around for years and has been perpetuated from one text book to another. In reality, the best way to protect the skin from the external environment is to 'waterproof' it so that it can defend itself. The use of talcum powder has little value in this. No matter how fine a talcum powder is, it will tend to clog and form itself into little granules in folds of skin like the toe webs, causing abrasion. If two surfaces are to glide smoothly over each other, this is best achieved by polishing the surfaces. Adequate moisturising not only waterproofs but also facilitates the smoothness of one surface gliding over the other.

A hair dryer is the best way to dry hair

Hair is in good condition when the cuticle cells on the hair shaft are tightly packed on top of each other and the outer surface is coated with an extremely thin layer of grease or sebum. When this is the case, individual hair shafts are waterproofed and shiny, and water from washing the hair should run off like 'water off a duck's back'. It should also dry easily with the aid of a towel or chamois dryer. Where a hair dryer is used on hair that is already damaged by over-shampooing, the exposed hair shaft can become vulnerable to extra weathering. Hence, while the occasional use of a hair dryer on healthy hair is not likely to cause too many problems, over-use on hair that has had its protection washed away by the overuse of shampoos could just cause more harm than good.

Expensive anti-wrinkle and rejuvenating creams do as they claim

The quest for eternal youth and beauty have been with us since time immemorial. And this has led to interest in any product that claims to have an effect on reducing aging. Wrinkles are a sign of skin aging (although they often result from excessive exposure to the sun rather than just to chronological age), and hence treatments claiming to eradicate wrinkles are likely to be much sought after. In recent times, treatments using retinol and vitamin A have been claimed to have this effect. They do so by causing a slight inflammation of the skin which causes a swelling and puffing so that wrinkles no longer show. Unfortunately, in causing inflammation these treatments also cause a redness of the skin, which is naturally not very popular. New creams that have attempted to overcome this effect tend to be made up of more and more complicated chemicals, and hence have the added danger of allergic reaction. To date, there are no effective anti-aging creams or medications without serious or unacceptable side effects.

The warmer you are in bed the better you sleep

This is akin to the belief that heavy snorers are better sleepers. Yet snoring is caused by an occlusion of the air passages. Sleep apnoea may be a part of this. Far from being a good sleeper, the snorer often suffers from daytime tiredness as a result of interrupted sleep during the night due to overheating and an inadequate oxygen

Why athletes who shave their legs could perform worse

Body hair serves the important function of trapping sweat and preventing it from falling off the body where its cooling function, through condensation on the skin, is wasted. The trend of some modern endurance athletes (other than swimmers) to shave their legs for aesthetic purposes could potentially impair performance by reducing the body's ability to cool itself when body temperatures are raised through the exertion of the exercise. Maintenance of body temperature with swimmers is not an issue because this is kept cool by the watery environment.

supply. Similarly, the notion of sleeping better while warmer can become counterproductive, as explained in Chapter 6. Indeed, overheating at night is one of the most common causes of poor quality sleep and of consequent skin problems, as we have regularly pointed out.

Exfoliating the skin helps to rejuvenate it

For many years, people have felt that by peeling off the outer layers of skin we can rejuvenate it. Peeling in the past was done using a range of chemicals from resorcinol to phenol and trichloroacetic acid. And while some of these, if skilfully used, can have some benefit, they can also produce problems with increased sensitivity to sunlight, scarring and disorders of pigmentation. Dr Aron-Brunetiere, the famous French dermatologist who has probably done more facial peels over the past 40 years than anyone else, claimed he would never do a peel in Europe between the months

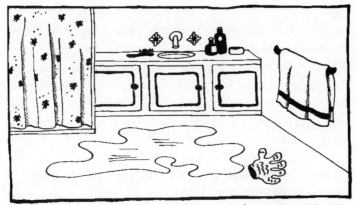

THE REMAINS OF DORIS PLATER WHO THOUGHT THAT SINCE THERE ARE SEVEN LAYERS OF SKIN SHE COULD LOSE WEIGHT BY EXFOLIATING THE FIRST SIX.

of April and September because of the problems with sunlight. He also claimed that he would never perform one in Australia because of the general exposure to sunlight all year round.

There has been a rise in the use of alpha hydroxy acids (AHAs) over the past twenty years in a vast number of everyday cosmetics, particularly in the United States where they are used quite indiscriminately. This has given rise to an ongoing investigation by the Food and Drug Administration (FDA), and the outcome of this is awaited with interest.

Most itchy eyes are caused by make-up

In a series of patients with itchy eyes investigated some years ago, only a small number were found to have positive patch tests to eye make-up and the author was left unsure of the cause.

A positive patch test does not necessarily mean that the chemical involved is the cause or the perpetuating factor. It may be like a footprint in the sand indicating that something has been there in the past, but may at this stage may no longer be involved. A patch test can also stay positive for most of one's life, although contact with the cause may have long passed. The results of heat studies show that eye rubbing occurs in people who are overheated at night and this is likely to be the most common cause of itchy eyes. Vigorous rubbing can probably also cause irritation of the conjunctiva, and even recurring damage to the cornea. Such conditions are not necessarily allergic or infective.

Collagen and elastin can be restored to the skin through creams or lotions

Collagen is one of the chemicals which helps bind skin together. Elastin is responsible for the elasticity in the dermis. With aging, both collagen and elastin decrease in effectiveness. This can be demonstrated by pinching a fold of skin on the back of the hand and watching to see how quickly this returns to normal. In a young person (i.e. less than twenty), the skin will 'bounce back' quickly. In an older person, or in someone who has experienced skin aging through exposure to sunlight, the skin will stay 'pinched' and only slowly return to its original form.

If collagen and elastin could somehow miraculously be restored in aged skin this would prevent the appearance of aging and help to provide a form of rejuvenation. In fact, this is what many commercial skin care products claim. By supposedly including collagen and elastin in their formulation, they deceive consumers into believing that this will result in skin revitalisation. However, even if such substances were able to reach the bloodstream, it is doubtful they could be used to replace or replenish the existing material. The only real effect appears to be on the wallet—and even this effect is negative! Both collagen and elastin need to be produced in the skin by the fibroblast cells.

Certain foods are good for the skin

There are many myths associating certain foods with specific skin conditions e.g. chocolate with acne, and urticaria (hives) with foods such as seafood. These associations have generally been disproved. There is also no specific food that is good for the skin. The best diet for skin is a wide variety of different foods without excessive fat. This is not to deny that some people do have allergies and well documented adverse reactions to certain foods. However, these cases are in reality quite rare. In these circumstances medical treatment is needed to definitively diagnose the allergy and to provide appropriate treatment.

Putting moisturising creams on the face can cause comedones (blackheads or whiteheads), or excessive hair growth

There is no scientific basis for this. Many women in particular do not adequately moisturise their faces because they feel they have 'greasy' faces. In fact it can be shown that in many cases, people who complain about having a greasy face have some thick, tacky emulsion on the surface composed of sebum and sweat. Below this, however, the stratum corneum often tends to be dry and is likely to benefit from moisturiser. Far from causing a greasy face, moisturising creams are more likely to help solve the problem.

Moisturisers such as sorbolene can cause cancer

This story often does the rounds in beauty/cosmetics circles, despite the fact that there is no evidence to support it. Simple moisturisers and water soluble paraffins are almost inert, in contrast to more chemically based and even 'natural' products, which can contain a multiplicity of chemicals, any one of which can cause adverse reactions. Even vitamin E cream, which is often recommended as a moisturiser, is of dubious benefit when applied to the skin, but may cause severe allergic reactions.

Cold hands and feet are a sign of poor circulation

In the absence of definitive signs of poor skin or nail nutrition, this is not true. All the acral areas—fingers, toes, ear lobes and nose tip—should feel colder than the forehead, unless the body is trying to lose heat because of a fever or overheating. Cold hands and feet usually mean that the TRM is working well, but the internal thermostat may be poorly adjusted.

Proper skin care costs lots of money and time

The suggestions put forward in this book involve the use of inexpensive, over-the-counter preparations, all of which are safe and easily obtainable, coupled with a parcel of lifestyle changes that are most likely to benefit the skin. Most patients report that after an initial period of practice of this regime, they spend about half the time they previously spent in the bathroom. A summary of these recommended changes is included as the last chapter of this book.

10 A skin care package for the 21st century

We've covered a lot of different skin care facts to this point, many of which might contradict some well held ideas and rules. The purpose of this final chapter is to bring together those facts as succinctly as possible to provide a sensible, simple and affordable skin care program which is uninvasive and unintrusive. The underlying principle is to allow the skin to be its own master and operate under its optimal level of efficiency.

As mentioned throughout the book, all the skin care techniques discussed here should be seen as a package, and not in isolation from each other. If only some suggestions are taken up and the rest ignored, the results are less likely to be totally satisfactory. All of the recommendations should be undertaken together from the start. It must also be realised that this is unlikely to provide an overnight remedy (and in reality, nothing will). Patience and perseverance are necessary. An effective outcome can take at least three to four months, but the long-term results are worth the wait.

Showering/bathing
- Dry skin will be upset and made more irritable by overheating, overwashing and contact with garments made of wool or brushed nylon. If the skin is irritable, no soap should be used and oatmeal baths should be substituted.

- Moisturising cream mixed with water may be used as soap. It will adequately clean ALL areas of the skin.
- Keeping soap to a minimum will reduce the need for deodorants, which themselves can have a damaging effect on the skin.
- Showers may be taken as often as desired, but they should be brief and tepid. Very hot water should be avoided. Soap should be kept to an *absolute minimum*, and should be simple in type and not 'medicated'. Soap should be rinsed off well before patting dry.
- Avoid spa baths and other heat treatments such as saunas.
- Avoid bubble baths or bath salts and do not use antiseptics such as Dettol in the bath water, especially for children.
- If desired, use an oatmeal bath (not oatmeal soap) by doing the following:
  1. Put one cup of rolled oats in an old nylon stocking or muslin bag.
  2. Fill a bath with tepid water so the whole body can be immersed.
  3. Swish bag around in the water until it goes white.
  4. Soak in the bath and squeeze bag against inflamed skin (10–15 mins).
  5. After the bath, pat the skin dry gently.

Drying

- After each shower, half dry the skin by patting, rather than rubbing.
- Soak up most of the moisture from the hair with a chamois or absorbent towel.
- It is not necessary to have the skin completely dry.

Moisturising

- Use a simple, inexpensive moisturiser (such as sorbolene cream with glycerine), purchased from your chemist or supermarket, regularly after showering or washing.
- Half dry the skin by patting before applying moisturiser.
- Take approximately one teaspoon of moisturising cream and four teaspoonsful of water. Mix these well in the hands until a nice simple lotion is formed and then rub this all over the body.
- Since the cream neither smells nor stains (except on silk) and washes out of clothing by the normal means, it is unnecessary to wait for the skin to dry before dressing. (Some people prefer to rush around in the nude, making the beds etc., while the moisturiser dries into the skin, before dressing!) You may feel a little 'damp' or even 'sticky', but you will become accustomed to this, and the moisturiser will dry into the skin over the next twenty minutes or so. It is not necessary to wait until the body is totally dry.

Note: Occasionally when very dry skin is being moisturised, small red spots, some with minute pustules in the centre, may develop, especially on the thighs and forearms due to blockage of hair follicles. Such spots should be ignored. They are not infectious. Squeezing or rubbing will make them worse.

Clothing

- Aim to keep yourself comfortably cool both during the day and at night. If you feel cold, wait for a few minutes before putting on extra clothing. When the body is warmed up enough, consider taking off some clothing. After some weeks of doing this the body adjusts, and it becomes easier to cope with temperature changes.

- Punch holes in the insteps of hot shoes to enable them to 'breathe' as you walk.

Sports clothing

- Avoid synthetic, full body clothing such as lycra. Wear light cotton clothing that 'breathes' to allow sweat to be evaporated off the body.
- Do not overdress. There is no such thing as 'sweating weight off' by overdressing during exercise.
- Where possible keep the extremities such as arms and legs and the midriff bare to allow for maximum temperature equilibration and allow sweat evaporation.
- Wear chunky acrylic socks during exercise to 'wick away' moisture from overheated sweaty feet.

Hair care

- Avoid shampoos. Use one to two tablespoons of hair conditioner for washing hair.
- Avoid the frequent use of hair dryers, especially if these are on the hottest setting.

Skin care

- Avoid the use of aftershave, toners, tonics, astringents and cleansers.
- Do not try to exfoliate the skin—particularly if exposure to sunlight is imminent.
- Avoid chemicals and the overuse of antiseptics and 'medicated' skin care items.
- Use moisturising cream as 'soap', hand cream, shaving cream, facial cleanser, moisturiser and shampoo if desired

(mix with a little water and rub into the scalp at night, then rinse out the next day).

- Reduce body fat (not necessarily weight).
- Reduce the amount of chemicals (in cosmetics products) applied to the skin.
- Don't be fooled by cosmetics that claim to be 'natural'.
- Use basic lipsticks/lip balms for moisturising and protecting the lips.
- Learn techniques of stress management.

Indoors

- Where possible, avoid situations of constant over-heating. To move from an airconditioned office to an airconditioned car to a heated home means the body is never required to adjust to normal temperature variations. In the meantime, the skin will dry out and become more exposed to the insults of the natural and imposed environments.
- Avoid rubber gloves while washing up.
- Don't use excessive detergent in the washing up. Using enough to form about twelve bubbles is usually sufficient.
- Use a bowl of water to increase humidity in an air-conditioned office.
- Take frequent breaks outdoors.

Outdoors

- Use a maximum protection sunscreen at all times if exposed to the sun.
- Move around if it is necessary to stay in the sun. Do not sunbake.

- Use sun protective clothing if exposed to the sun over long periods.
- Regularly wear a sun protective hat.
- Use moisturiser after sun and salt water or chlorine exposure.
- Wear sunglasses when in the outdoors, but choose a brand based on UV protection level (preferably 100 per cent) rather than on price.

Night-time

- Use blankets and sheets instead of a doona or quilt.
- Avoid electric blankets or heated waterbeds.
- Use light, natural fibre blankets such as wool (but not angora or mohair).
- Go 'cold turkey' by having about ten consecutive cool nights. In spring and autumn this involves sleeping with only one cotton sheet. In winter it should be done with one sheet and one cotton or wool blanket. Frequent waking may occur in the first few nights but better sleep usually occurs after about a week.
- Do not use bed socks.
- If cold feet are a problem, heat a towel in a microwave for two to three minutes, and place under the feet. (Don't burn the hands picking up very hot towels.)
- Avoid the use of hot-water bottles.
- Wear light night attire all year round.

Travelling

- If possible, in a hotel/motel room, turn off the air-conditioning and open the window. If this is not possible, half fill the bath with water and leave overnight.

- If spending long periods in an airconditioned or heated car, use a light spray mist to increase the humidity.
- Carry a moisturiser in hand luggage for use on long-distance airplane flights.
- Ask the hotel if it is possible to have blankets instead of a doona or continental quilt.

Baby skin care

- Avoid the use of 'skin wipes' etc. on baby skin. They often contain disguised detergents/grease solvents etc., leading to overcleansing.
- Ensure that the baby does not spend hours in bed in a soaked nappy. Nappies should be changed about two hours after the last feed. This can often be done without waking the child.
- Substitute any simple inert moisturiser (i.e. vaseline, zinc and cod liver oil, sorbolene with 10 per cent glycerine) for talcum powder. They are all good for keeping the skin well waterproofed and protected.
- It is important to avoid overheating at all times, especially at night. Typically, the overheated child will kick off the bed covers, trying to send a message to the parents that they are too hot. This message will be repeated. Some parents refuse to receive it. Overdressing during the day can have unwanted effects on both skin and temperature.
- Occasionally nappy rashes can be complicated by an overgrowth of monilia, especially if the baby has been on antibiotics. This can make the rash difficult to clear. Medical advice should be sought. A short course of Nystatin by mouth may be helpful.

Summary

The skin is an effective signalling organ which represents the barrier between what is going on 'inside' and 'outside' the body. As such, it is exposed to a range of 'insults' ranging from internal psychological causes to the external environment. This book has not considered the internal causes to any great extent, but instead has concentrated on those external, environmental causes that are often neglected in cosmetic approaches to skin care. In the main, these are dryness, overcleansing and inappropriate skin treatments. And while these conclusions are far from startling, it is to be hoped that they can provide a new way of looking at skin care which will give benefit to those many people for whom it has been a problem in the past.

Index